T0135799

Nina Trukhacheva

Modern Methods
of Statistical Analysis of Medical Data

Logos Verlag Berlin

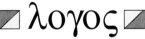

Bibliographic information published by the Deutsche Nationalbibliothek

The Deutsche Nationalbibliothek lists this publication in the Deutsche
Nationalbibliografie; detailed bibliographic data are available
in the Internet at http://dnb.d-nb.de .

ISBN 978-3-8325-3818-7

Logos Verlag Berlin GmbH
Comeniushof, Gubener Str. 47,
10243 Berlin
Tel.: +49 (0)30 42 85 10 90
Fax: +49 (0)30 42 85 10 92
INTERNET: http://www.logos-verlag.de

ANNOTATION

The monograph "Modern Methods of Statistical Analysis of Medical Data" covers both parametric and non-parametric methods of analysis which are considered to be fundamental: descriptive statistics, analysis of variance and relations, multiple regression analysis as well as modern methods such as factor analysis, discriminant analysis, cluster analysis and loglinear analysis. Most books on biostatistics can be divided into two categories: first group of books applies academic mathematical approaches which do not give a clear understanding to medics; the second group is based on simplified mathematical apparatus without explanations of basic principles. This book is among the few where the author strictly but perfectly clear describes the principles of each method providing scheme of its application and indicating possible limitations and errors.

The book consists of two parts. The first part outlines the theoretical basis of biostatistics. It determines fundamental concepts which are used for planning the statistical analysis. The research material for statistical processing should be prepared correctly to get the reliable results. For competent statistical analysis the task should be formulated in such a way that appropriate statistical methods can be applied for it solution, in other words, a mathematical and statistical model should be developed.

It is the most difficult point of the working plan for beginners since they need to outline the opportunities given by applied statistics, and understand which of them can be useful for a particular purpose. Finally, it is important to consider what the data requirements accompany these methods, and verify whether these requirements are satisfied. The book provides the schemes which show a wide range of methods used to solve the most common tasks. Traditional textbooks usually focus on statistical conclusions based on the assumption of a normal distribution of variables, including multivariate statistical methods such as regression, factor and dispersion analyses. However, parametric methods cannot be used in every case, even for continuous variables, especially for a small sample. As regards practical tasks, they often require to identify the differences and relations of ordinal or discrete variables or a set of different variables. Taking into consideration these factors, the book covers non-parametric methods of data analysis.

However, the theory becomes clear and understandable if it can be used to solve practical tasks. Therefore, besides the theoretical fundamentals the second part of the text describes application of the software package Statistica for solving medical tasks which simplifies them and reduces task completion time. Such a choice is also connected with the convenience of export and import of data and results in this system. Solving tasks are considered step by step. The text is well illustrated with pictures and screenshots which are extremely helpful in acquiring skills to use theoretical knowledge in practice. The author had to sacrifice strict mathematical descriptions in order to make the text clear for a wide range of readers. Cumbersome proving is replaced by simple and not very strict explanation. All examples are taken from clinical practice or developed hypothetically to illustrate the method briefly. For some readers too many details may seem to be the disadvantage. However, due to minute description the text can solve problems with minimal loss of time. It is up to the reader to decide whether it is good or bad.

The book is intended primarily for medical students and health care professionals who are more interested in applying statistical methods than their strict mathematical justification. It will be useful for practicing physicians and researchers to critically evaluate the medical literature and planning, conducting and analyzing the results of research. However, it may be useful as an introductory course for those who want to study biostatistics more profoundly. This book will give an opportunity to get a clear understanding of biostatistics, its methods and the place occupied in medical education and work of the practicing physicians.

To my mother Anna Trukhacheva

INTRODUCTION

The monograph presents the revised and corrected lectures given by the author to students and researchers of Altai State Medical University. It focuses on the fundamentals of biostatistics for medical data analyzing. Each theory becomes more understandable and accessible, if it is possible to use it for solution of practical problems. For this reason the monograph describes how to solve problems using the software package Statistica in addition to theoretical basics. It allows every interested reader to acquire skills of using theoretical knowledge in practice, and makes the tasks solution significantly faster. The author had to sacrifice strict mathematical descriptions in order to make the text clear for a wide range of readers. Cumbersome proving is replaced by simple and not very strict explanation. All examples are taken from clinical practice or developed hypothetically to illustrate the method briefly. For some readers too many details may seem to be the disadvantage. However, due to minute description the text can solve problems with minimal loss of time. It is up to the reader to decide whether it is good or bad.

The book is intended primarily for medical students and health care professionals who are more interested in applying statistical methods than their strict mathematical justification. It will be useful for practicing physicians and researchers to critically evaluate the medical literature and planning, conducting and analyzing the results of research. However, it may be useful as an introductory course for those who want to study biostatistics more profoundly.

I sincerely appreciate the assistance of people who helped me with the monograph. I express my profound gratitude for support and discussion of this work to Professor Yu. A. Vysotskij, Dr. N.P. Pupyrev and Dr. S.V.Hlybova. I thank tremendously for the design E.I.Vorsin and M. V. Nechaev.

N. Trukhacheva

CHAPTER 1

HISTORY OF BIOSTATISTICS

The history of statistical science is said to start in the middle of the XVIII century; although the practical operations to collect data on population, its structure, property status, and other information were known long before. The term "statistics" derived from the Latin *status* designating "state of affairs". Originally statistics described the "sights" of the state, and only in the XIX century statistical information was started to be quantified.

Statistical science is associated with names of English economist William Petty (1623-1687) and John Graunt (1629-1674) whose statistical and demographic ideas were developed by their followers - German pastor Johann Peter Sussmilch II (1707-1767) and the prominent Belgian scientist of the XIX century Lambert-Adolph-Jacques Quetelet (1796-1874). Adolph Quetelet's works showed the importance of statistics in learning laws of social life, detecting that these laws are clearly evident only in the mass of phenomena; that is, studying data on a large number of cases. In addition A. Quetelet founded biometrics. His doctrine of statistical regularity was developed by German statistician and economist William Lexis (1837-1914).

Further development of statistical science is associated with works of Francis Galton (1822-1911), Karl Pearson (1857-1936), Ronald Fisher (1890-1962), William Sealy Gosset (1876-1937) and other Western scholars. A number of indicators and criteria were named after them. F. Galton introduced the term "regression" in 1886. He found out that on average children of tall fathers are not so tall, and sons of fathers of small stature are taller than their fathers. This was interpreted by him as "regression towards mediocrity." K. Pearson improved the methods of correlation and regression proposed by F. Galton. K. Pearson introduced to statistics such concepts as standard deviation and variation. He developed chi-squared test and introduced generally accepted term "normal distribution". The idea of controlled clinical trials appeared in the XII century when Frederick II, Holy Roman Emperor, studied how physical exercises influenced digestion. Two knights had been given the same food; then one of them went to bed, and the other went a-hunting. A few hours later he killed both of them and made a careful study of their digestive tracts. Digestion of the sleeping man was more intensive. In the XVII century Jan Baptist van Helmont decided to call into question the practice of bloodletting and offered the first randomized clinical trial with a large number of participants and statistical analysis. About 500 people were expected to be randomly divided into two groups. Bloodletting was not used in one of the group. As regards the other group, doctors could apply this method as many times as it was necessary. The effectiveness of bloodletting was evaluated due to the number of funerals in each group. For unknown reasons the experiment was not carried out; however, later bloodletting was proved to be ineffective by P. Louis.

However, extensive use of statistical data for medical research was started only in the XIX century. The science of application of mathematics in biology directly intertwined with the development of genetics. It was genetics, and especially Mendel's Genetic Laws, to become the main area of application of statistical methods in biology. Recently statistical methods having penetrated into different branches of medicine have become the principal methods of analysis and processing of the experimental data. However, power of developed statistical research methods tend to come into conflict with the lack of adequate knowledge of doctors who have to use these methods. Any doctor should be familiar with the basic principles and methods of statistics in order to competently discuss new diagnostic techniques and choose the best method of treatment. German scholar H.G. Wells pointed out that not only doctors but any modern person should have such a "statistical thinking":"Statistisches Denken wird für den mündigen Bürger eines Tages dieselbe Bedeutung haben wie die Fähigkeit, lesen und schreiben zu können". Due to the wide spreading of the "evidence based medicine" ideology in the world, recently the fundamentals of biostatistics have become a necessary element of education at the medical schools.

CHAPTER 2

DESCRIPTIVE STATISTICS

2.1. RANDOM EVENTS AND RANDOM VARIABLES

When studying one's health, it is essential to consider many factors - both improving and worsening one's medical condition. All these factors must be expressed in certain quantitative estimations. To obtain necessary numerical data, a number of observations is required, as most of the random and unforeseen events are subjected to some general non-random laws.

The science that studies the pattern of mass random events is called the theory of probability. Application of the probability theory to the processing of a large set of numbers is called mathematical statistics.

The examples of random events are everywhere. For instance, in questions: "Will it snow tomorrow? Which side will a tossed up coin fall down?" In other words, whenever there is no complete information, an accident occurs.

Statistical definition of probability

Ratio limit of the number of trials m, in which the event A happened, to the total number of trials n, providing that the total number of trials n goes to infinity, is called probability of the event A.

$$P(A) = \lim_{n \to \infty} \frac{m}{n}$$

The number of trials must be large enough. For instance, two trials are insufficient to determine the probability of appearance of heads or tails, as in each of the cases both heads and tails can appear. Therefore the probability of their appearance will be 100%.

The definition of probability given above is named statistical. It allows calculating the probability of such events, the structure of which is unknown and the frequency of which cannot be predicted in advance. For example, only the statistical data collected over the years made it possible to find the boys and girls birth probability. It turned out that these probabilities are different. The boys' birth probability is about 0.52; therefore, the girls birth probability is 0.48.

THE NOTION OF RANDOM VARIABLE

Random variable is a variable whose value is subject to variations due to chance and cannot be predicted on the basis of trial conditions.

Even the most accurate method of analysis gives certain deviation in the results when repeated (repeatability error). It means that every numerical result is a random event. Sugar and hormones content in blood, height and weight etc. of a patient under examination are all random. In medicine and biology the patient is regarded as an *object* of observation. During the observations severity of illness, height, weight, quantitative data of laboratory assessment etc. are defined. Certain parameters such as gender are qualitative; others such as height are quantitative.

Random variables can be divided into two basic classes: *discrete and continuous*.

- **Discrete** random variables take on strictly defined values and there can be no other values between them.
- **Continuous** random variables take on any value within a given interval.

THE TYPES OF SCALES IN STATISTICS (OR TYPES OF VARIABLES)

Variables differ by how "precise" they can be measured or, in other words, how much measureable information is provided by their measurement scale. Type of the scale, in which the measurement is performed, is another factor that determines the amount of information which variable contains. The following types of scales are distinguished: *nominal scale, ordinal scale, interval scale, and ratio scale.*

  – **Nominal scale** is used only for proper objects classification in order to distinguish one object from another: number of an animal in the group or the unique code assigned to him, etc. Such variables can be measured only in reference to different classes; however, these classes cannot be arranged. Typical examples of nominal variables are gender, nationality, color etc. Nominal variables are also known as *categorical*. Categorical variables are often presented as the monitoring frequency referred to specific categories and classes. If there are only two classes, the variable is called *dichotomous*. For example: 1 – male gender, 2 – female gender. It is seen that coding of the variable *gender* with the help of numbers 1 and 2 is absolutely arbitrary; they could be interchanged or represented with another numbers. The same situation is with the variable *marital status*. In this case again the correspondence between the numbers and categories of marital status has no empirical value. But in contrast to gender, this variable is not dichotomous – it has four code numbers instead of two: 1 – single, 2 – married, 3 – widower/widow, 4 – divorced. Processing capabilities of nominal scale variables are very limited. For instance, the calculation of mean value for the variable *gender* is completely pointless.

  – **Ordinal scale.** This scale only arranges objects assigning to them various grades. In addition it indicates which of them to a greater or lesser extent possess the quality evaluated by the variable. However, values of the variables do not provide the possibility to say "how much bigger" or "how much smaller" one value is than another. Numbers of buildings on the streets are measured in ordinal scale. A typical example of an ordinal variable – clothing size: S, M, L, XL, XXL, XXXL, XXXXL. The Mohs scale of mineral hardness is also ordinal. School grading scale (five points, twelve points, etc.) can be attributed to the ordinal scale. Variable *Smoking* is possible to rank on an ordinal scale from the bottom upwards: 1- do not smoke, 2 – smoke rarely, 3 – smoke often, 4 – smoke very often. Light smoker smokes more than non-smoker, while heavy smoker smokes more than light smoker, etc. The scale of hypertensive disease stages, heart failure degrees scale, scale of coronary insufficiency stages are ordinal scales in medicine. In this case comparing mean values in two samplings makes no sense. The empirical importance of these variables does not depend on the difference between the neighboring numerical values. Thus, despite the fact that the difference between the values of code numbers for non-smoker, light smoker and heavy smoker in both cases equals one, it is impossible to say that the actual difference between non-smoker, light smoker and heavy smoker is the same. These concepts are too vague to draw such conclusions.

  – **Interval scale** not only allows arranging the measurement objects, but also makes it possible to express them numerically and compare the difference between them. For example, the temperature, measured in the degrees Fahrenheit or degrees Celsius, generates the interval scale. According to the Celsius scale, as it is known, 0°C was defined as the freezing point of water and 100°C was defined as the boiling point of water. Consequently, the temperatures interval between the freezing point and the boiling point is divided into 100 equal parts. In this case it will be wrong to declare that a body with a temperature of 40°C is two times hotter than a body with a temperature of 20°C. The interval scale keeps the length ratio of the intervals. It is not only possible to say that the temperature of 40°C is higher than the temperature of 30°C, but also that the increase of temperature from 20°C up to 40°C is twice as high as the increase from 30°C up to 40°C. Now consider the intelligence quotient (IQ). Its absolute values show ordinal relation between the respondents, and the difference between the two values is also empirically important. For example, if Fedor's IQ is 80, Peter's is 120 and Ivan's is 160, it is possible to say that Peter is as "intelligent" in comparison to Fedor as Ivan is "intelligent" in comparison to Peter (i.e. – by 40 units). However, it is impossible to conclude that Ivan is twice smarter than Fedor based only on the fact that Fedor's IQ is two times smaller. Such variables can be processed with any statistical methods without restrictions. It means, for instance, that a mean value is a valid statistical indicator to characterize such variables.

- **Ratio scale** measures almost all physical quantities - time, linear dimensions, areas, volumes, current strength, power, etc. This is the most powerful scale. This scale includes all the interval variables that have an absolute zero point. For example, the Kelvin temperature scale forms the ration scale, and it can be asserted that a body with a temperature of 200°K is twice hotter than a body with a temperature of 100°K. Age can become the example of the variable referred to the ratio scale: if Andrew is 30, and Alex is 60, we can say that Alex is two times elder than Andrew.

Ratio scale will take place in biomedical research when time of appearance of criteria after beginning of action (time threshold in seconds, minutes), intensity of action before appearance of any criteria (action force threshold in volts, x-rays, etc.). Ration scales includes all the data in biochemical and electrophysiological research (concentration of substances, time indices of electrocardiogram etc.). For example, the number of correctly or incorrectly performed "tasks" in various tests studying higher nervous activity of animals is also referred to ration scales. Note that most statistical procedures do not distinguish the properties of interval scales and ratio scales. Mean value, standard deviation can be calculated for the latter two scales.

In practice, including the data processing with the Statistica software package, the difference between the variables related to the interval scale and ratio scale, is usually unimportant. It is possible to shift from more powerful scale to the weaker one. Thus, the continuous variables can be categorized. For example, the continuous random variable *height* can be shifted from the ration scale into ordinal scale with gradations: short, low, medium and high.

However, it should be taken into consideration that the transition to the nominal scale from the scales of the higher order, we lose some information about the observations. Observations that differed from each other within the interval scale can be perceived as equal within the nominal scale. Therefore it is recommended to apply the nominal scale only when there is no any opportunity to use a scale of the higher order.

PARENT POPULATION AND SAMPLE
RANDOM DISTRIBUTION

The main method of testing in biostatistics is sampling. In its most general form it looks the following way: there is a large set of *N* objects which is called ***parent population***. As a rule, ***parent population*** is only imaginary, hypothetical complete collection of objects (people, animals, plants or things) which is a source of the data.

The *n* objects are derived from the set that form the ***sample*** (***sample is a part of the population obtained for the study***); the number *n* is called sample size. These *n* objects are studied in details. Due to the results of the research, it is required to describe the entire population or any of its properties and characteristics.

The sampling method is used in the study of seed germination, within different demographic and economic research, for control of production and in medical research. At first sight, this method is not much different from the ordinary method of small samples. For example, within the analysis of a substance, all studies are conducted over small amounts (samples) of the substance. However, the difference is very significant. Analyzing the substance, we certainly know that the criterion we are interested in (number of various ions) is distributed uniformly throughout the substance, and, therefore, any small sample is a true copy of the whole substance. Within the frames of the sampling method studied criterion is distributed unevenly in the parent population, and even the nature of the unevenness is unknown. Therefore, not every sample reflect the structure of the whole population in a proper way. Imagine that you want to study the average height of a population of the city, and you are offered the basketball team as a sample. It is easy to understand how the result will be distorted.

Having no information about the parent population and making the selection, we can only rely on chance - all other methods of selection will be biased bearing the traces of extraneous factors. *All objects must be selected completely in a random manner.* The situation is different if we know in advance that the parent population consists of several classes which are different in their characteristics. Under these conditions, it is better to collect random sample from each class independently. For example, studying the height of people, separate samples of men and women are collected. Sometimes age, profession and place of residence are taken into account.

Sample which reflects properties of the population is called ***representative.***

The random nature of the sample implies that any judgment on the parent population due to the sample is random itself.

Set of allowed values x_i very poorly characterizes a random variable. In order to fully characterize a random variable, and even to make further predictions, it is necessary not only to specify which values xi can possess, but also how often it takes on these values. In other words, it is necessary to set the distribution of this random variable.

METHODS OF RANDOM VARIABLES ASSIGNMENT

Description of the set of values of the random variable indicating the probability of each value is called *distribution law of a variable.*

More generally, to set the distribution law of a discrete random variable, it is necessary just to write down all its values, and corresponding *frequency* P_i (or frequency of occurrence m_i) for each of them. Usually such record is made as a table where the top line shows the value of a random variable, and the bottom line -the probabilities of these values (or frequency of occurrence m_i). The resulting table is called distribution law of a random variable. This type of assignment of a random variable called tabular.

After receiving the sample, all its objects are examined in relation to a certain random variable – i.e. to the characteristics of the object which are under consideration. It results in the observed data which represents a set of numbers arranged out of order. This set of data is usually called statistical series. The analysis of such data is very difficult, and the received data are ranked to study the patterns.

Example 2.1 According to the observation performed by health workers, the pulse rate of 25 boys from the kindergarten was the following number of beats per second:

$$74,70,70,74,68,68,66,78,76,70,74,76,82,80,74,65,69,71,69,68,72,71,73,72,70$$

Discrete values of a random variable after ranking are arranged in ascending or descending order. After ranking the experimental data are combined in such a manner that the values of a random variable in each group are the same. The value of a random variable corresponding to a particular group of the integrated set of the observed data, is called *variant*, and value change is called variation. Variants will be denoted by letters with the corresponding serial number of indices $x_1, x_2, ..., x_n$, where n – number of groups. Meanwhile, $x_1 < x_2 < ... < x_n$.

The number of a separate group of the integrated set of data is called frequency m_i, where i – index of the variant, and the ratio of frequency of this variant to the total sum of frequencies is called *relative frequency* and is denoted p:

$$p = \frac{m_i}{n},$$

$i = 1, ..., n$, i.e.

$$\frac{m_i}{n} = \frac{m_i}{\sum_{i=1}^{m} m_i}.$$

Discrete variation series is a ranged set of variants x_i with the corresponding frequencies m_i or quotient $\frac{m_i}{n}$. *Statistical series arranged in ascending or descending order is called a variation series* .

As the result of the above mentioned operations thirteen values of the random variables have been received, each of them is found a certain value of times. Thus, the discrete series is obtained which shows the calculated values of the frequencies and relative frequencies:

Table 2-2

Variation series

Variant x_i	65	66	68	69	70	71	72	73	74	76	78	80	82
Frequency m_i	1	1	3	2	4	2	2	1	4	2	1	1	1
Relative frequency $\dfrac{m_i}{n}$	0.04	0.04	0.12	0.08	0.16	0.08	0.08	0.04	0.16	0.08	0.04	0.04	0.04

In contrast to the initial data, this series allows making some conclusions about the statistical regularities.

If the number of possible values of a discrete random variable is quite large or the observed random variable is continuous, the interval variation series is constructed, which is understood as an ordered population of variability intervals of the values of a random variable with the corresponding frequencies or relative frequencies of being within the each value of the random variable.

As a rule, subintervals which make the entire range of variation have the same length and can be represented as

$$(x_i, x_i + \Delta x), \quad i = 1, 2, ..., k,$$

where k – number of intervals.

The length Δx should be chosen in such a manner to avoid the unhandiness of the constructed series but at the same time allows detecting changes of the random variable.

The following formula is recommended for Δx :

$$\Delta x = \frac{x_{\max} - x_{\min}}{k},$$

where x_{max}, x_{min} – maximum and minimum value of a random variable.

The number of intervals is calculated due to the *Sturges' formula*:

$$k = 1 + 3.322 \cdot \lg n.$$

If it is found that that Δx is a fractional number, then the length of the interval is taken as the nearest simple fraction, or the nearest integer value. Thus, it is necessary that the following conditions work:

$$x_1 \le x_{\min}; \quad x_k + \Delta x \ge x_{\max}.$$

After the particular intervals have been found, the number of values of the random variable within the given intervals are determined. The interval includes the value greater or equal to the lower boundary and smaller than the upper boundary. Reconstruct the discrete variation series from **Example 2.1** into the interval one.

Solution. Since the biggest variant is 82, and the smallest is 65, the entire sample is found within the interval (65, 82). According to the *Herbert Sturges' formula*, six subintervals are obtained. The length of each subinterval is $\dfrac{82 - 65}{6} \approx 3$.

The first interval has five values of the variable; the second - eight, etc.

The appropriate interval variational series is called grouped.

13

Table 2-3

Grouped interval variational series

X	65-68	68-71	71-74	74-77	77-80	80-83
m_i	5	8	7	2	2	1

Frequency polygons. Hystogram

The second method to define a random variable is *graphic*. The values of the discrete random variable, its frequencies and relative frequencies are plotted. If the points are joined, the plot in the shape of a broken line will be constructed which is called *polygon* (Figure 2.1).

In case of a grouped variational series for discrete and continuous random variable, the intervals of its values Δx_i, frequency m_i or relative frequency $P_i = \dfrac{m_i}{n}$ are plotted. Such a plot which is called a *histogram* will roughly reflect the distribution of the continuous random variable at the number axis (Fig. 2.2). If the intervals are equal, it is possible to construct a histogram in coordinates $x_i \leftrightarrow m_i$ or $x_i \leftrightarrow P_i$. If the intervals are not equal, the histogram is constructed in the coordinates $x_i \leftrightarrow f_i$, where f_i - probability density, the value describing the probability distribution within the interval.

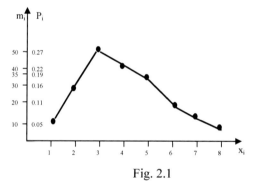

Fig. 2.1

Probability density is the ratio of the probability of a random variable occurrence to the interval of values with in which it occurs:

$$f_i = \frac{P_i}{\Delta x_i}.$$

It follows then: $P_i = f_i \Delta x_i$. i.e. probability is equal to the area of a rectangle with the height f_i and the width Δx_i (shaded area in Fig. 2.3).

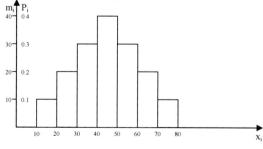

Fig. 2.2

Histogram and polygon roughly determine the distribution of the random variable. Histogram and polygon can be constructed for both discrete and continuous random variable. In practice more often polygon is constructed for a discrete random variable, and histogram- for a continuous random variable.

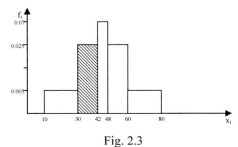

Fig. 2.3

Obviously, it is possible to assume that with the decrease of the width the plot will take the form of a smooth curve (Fig. 2.4), which, like any other curve can be represented as a formula, i.e. analytically.

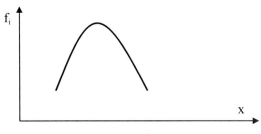

Fig. 2.4

Random variable distribution can be described analytically by different formulas. Depending on the formula and parameters it includes, the distribution can be called: the Poisson distribution, the Maxwell distribution, binomial distribution, exponential distribution, etc. The number of possible types of distributions is very large. However, in practice not many distributions are often used. The analysis of the various random variables, studied theoretically and calculated on the basis of experiments, demonstrates that one the most frequently found distribution is normal.

2.2. NORMAL DISTRIBUTION OF A RANDOM VARIABLE.

NUMERICAL CHARACTERISTICS OF NORMAL DISTRIBUTION AND THEIR POINT ESTIMATIONS

The distribution of a random variable is called *normal,* if the form of the distribution curve is described by the following formula:

$$f(x) = \frac{1}{\sqrt{2\pi}\sigma} e^{-\frac{(x-a)^2}{2\sigma^2}}.$$

This function is called *Gaussian (named after Carl Friedrich Gauß) probability-density function. Mathematical expectation a and standard deviation σ are the function's main parameters.* The bell, which is symmetric with respect to the distribution center, represents the normal distribution diagram.

As a rule, samples, which strictly obey *normal distribution,* do not occur in practice; while the distributions that do not purely meet the standards of normal distribution but having similarity with it frequently do. The similarities are due to the fact that extreme values of variations, close to x_{min} and $x_{max,}$ appear more rarely than medial. In practice, during primary data processing it is almost always necessary to clarify if the real distribution can be considered to be normal, and to what extent the defined distribution differs from *normal.* This can be done by means of tests for concordance.

The normal distribution has two attributes:

1. The farther from the center, the lower the branches of the graph are. This shows decrease in probability of the random variable appearance in case of its strong deviation from the central value.

2. The graph is symmetric about the center. This suggests that the appearance of the random variable's value is as possible to the right as it is to the left of the center.

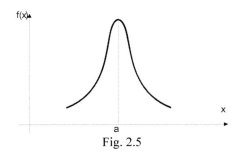

Fig. 2.5

Remember the formula $P_i = f_i \Delta x_i$. Let's break the graph into narrow intervals within which the probability density remains almost constant. Now it is easy to understand that probability equals the area S, $P = S!$

Gauss's formula includes two values. These values are *numerical characteristics of a random variable, or parameters of a random variable.* Their value determines the type of the distribution plot. Detecting and indicating these random variable parameters is challenging in mathematical statistics.

The first parameter is *mathematical expectation.* It is denoted by *a.* It characterizes the distribution center of a random variable. The formula

$$a = \sum x_i p_i \,,$$

where x_i – random variable values – height, weight, and etc., p_i – occurrence probability of the random variable values, is used to find mathematical expectation. Supposing that $P_i = \dfrac{m_i}{N}$, then

$$a = \dfrac{\sum\limits_{i=1}^{N} x_i m_i}{N} \,,$$

which shows that *mathematical expectation – is the mean value of the random variable within the population.* The plot shows that in case of $x = a$, the curve has a maximum. Thus, *mathematical expectation is the most frequent value of a random variable.* In medical and biological research mathematical expectation is defined as a true value.

Variance is another numerical characteristic of a random variable. It is denoted by letter D or σ^2 ($D = \sigma^2$). Variance represents the measure of the random variables values dispersion near the center of distribution. Some of the random variable values differ from the center more than others. To evaluate the degree of deviation of any random variable value from the center (from mathematical expectation), and in other words, to estimate average deviation, it is necessary to put together all deviations $(x_i - a)$ and divide by the number of trials.

But considering the fact that all deviations are equally probable for normal distribution, it is only possible to get zero answer, because the deviations to the left of the center are negative, and to the right − are positive.

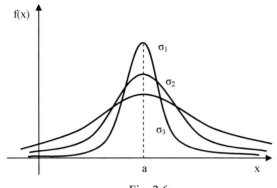

Fig. 2.6

The deviations have to be squared to avoid such situation. It results in the following formula:

$$D = \frac{\sum_{i=1}^{N}(x_i - a)^2 m_i}{N},$$

where N – the population size. Hence, the dispersion will have the dimension of a random variable, but only squared. It is required to extract the square root of the variance to get rid of such "inconvenience". Obviously, the value obtained from dispersion also characterizes the spread or dispersion of the random variable values around the center. The square root of variance is called the mean square deviation, or *standard deviation*, and is denoted by the letter σ ($\sigma = \sqrt{D}$); then

$$\sigma = \sqrt{\frac{\sum_{i=1}^{N}(x_i - a)^2 m_i}{N}}$$

When the parameter σ decreases, ordinate $f(x)$ of the curve increases. The rise of the curve in the central part is counterbalanced by the sharper decline to its axis 0x, so that the total area remains unchanged and equals to one $P = S = 1$. In Fig. 2.6 the plots with the same mathematical expectation but with different dispersion are shown.

In theory, the random variable distributed according to the normal law can take on any value from −∞ to +∞. In fact, as the plot demonstrates, the probability density rapidly decreases with distance from the center, and as $x = a \pm 3\sigma$, the probability density values can be neglected (Fig.2.7).

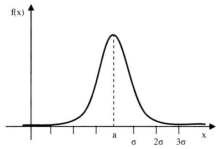

Fig. 2.7

17

Let's analyze the distribution graphs of men and women's life expectancy as an example. Both graphs refer to the normal distribution, though numerical characteristics of these distributions are different, so the graphs will differ (Fig. 2.8). It is known that women's average life expectancy is higher, so the graph will be shifted to the left on the number axis.

It's also a well-known fact that men, for various reasons (war, domestic conflicts, suicide, etc.) can die at an early age, but at the same time there are more long-livers who outlived average age among men then there are among women. Therefore, variance is higher for men, which means their graph will be wider, but lower, since the area which equals probability must be common and equal to one.

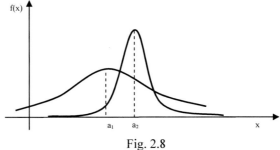

Fig. 2.8

Irrelevance to normal distribution can be caused not only by the specificity of characteristics variation, but also by qualitative nonhomogeneity of the sample. Fig. 2.9 represents a typical example of this sort. It illustrates the variability of characteristic in the sample of patients of different ages. The histogram clearly shows that the shape of the distribution has a double-humped appearance. The left peak of distribution corresponds to different age groups. Thus, incongruence with normal distribution, in this case, is clearly determined by the objects of study's age variability. In this and similar cases, it is more appropriate to divide the original sample into qualitatively more homogeneous groups.

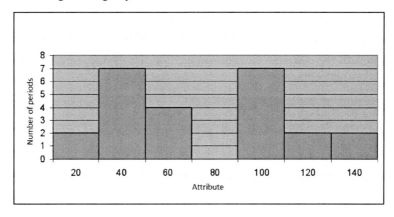

Fig. 2.9

POINT ESTIMATIONS OF THE POPULATION PARAMETERS DUE TO THE SAMPLES

The mean value, variance and standard deviation can be accurately calculated, if the data on every object of the population is available. Actually, it is rarely possible to examine all the objects of population. Usually, only sample is being studied, suggesting that the sample reflects the properties of the population. While analyzing the sample, the mean and standard deviation are not known for a certainty, but can be estimated. *Estimation* of the mean for population (i.e., mathematical expectation), calculated from a sample, is called *sample mean*. $\bar{x}$ stands for *sample mean* which is calculated by the formula:

$$\bar{x} = \frac{\sum_{i=1}^{n} x_i}{n},$$

where n – sample size.

Hence, $\bar{x} \approx a$. If characteristics' values have frequency, then the following formula should be used

$$\bar{x} = \frac{\sum_{i=1}^{n} x_i \cdot m_i}{\sum_{i=1}^{n} m_i}.$$

Estimation of the standard deviation is called *sample standard deviation* S_x and is evaluated as follows:

$$S_x = \sqrt{\frac{\sum_{i=1}^{n}(x_i - \bar{x})^2 m_i}{n-1}}.$$

This formula differs from the formula for the standard deviation of a population. First, mathematical expectation a is replaced by its sample estimation $\bar{x}$. Second, figure of one is subtracted from the number of sample members in the denominator. A rigorous substantiation of the latter statement requires a serious mathematical proof, but the following explanation would be quite enough here.   Internal scatter is never as great as in whole population, and the division on $n-1$ instead of n compensates the resulting underestimation of the standard deviation. I.e., if the denominator is $n-1$ instead of n, S_x more strictly corresponds to σ. It can be roughly written as $S_x \approx \sigma$.

The squared sample standard deviation is *sample variance D_x*.

$$D_x = S_x^2 \text{ or } D_x = \frac{\sum_{i=1}^{n}(x_i - \bar{x})^2}{n-1}.$$

Sample variance (also referred to as *corrected variance) makes an estimate* of the variance in the population $D_x \approx D$.

Sample arithmetical mean and standard deviation are estimations of the arithmetic mean and standard deviation for population calculated from the random sampling. It is possible to take several samples from one population. It is clear that different samples give different estimates. Consider, for example, the height of 200 students. Even if several samples are taken from the population, and an average height is calculated in each of them, the values, though being different, will not differ from each other significantly. In other words, their variance is smaller than the variance of an individual value (height value of a certain student). It is possible to notice that the set of 25 average samples, for instance, has bell curve distribution similar to normal one. Since the distribution is normal, it can be described by the mean value and standard deviation.

Since the mean value for 25 points under analysis is mean of the values which themselves are also average, it should be represented as $\bar{X}$. Similarly, $S_{\bar{x}}$ should stand for standard deviation of average values. Hence,

$$S_{\bar{x}} = \frac{S_x}{\sqrt{n}}.$$

The mean value of sample means $\overline{X}$ is equal to the average value of entire population of 200 students. Thus, the average value of sample means coincides with the average mean for the population (mathematical expectation a).

Just as standard deviation S_x of the original sample of 10 students is an evaluation of students' height variableness, $S_{\overline{x}}$ also is the evaluation of average values variableness of 25 samples with 10 students in each. Thus, the value $S_{\overline{x}}$ is a measure of the accuracy with which the sample mean is an estimate of the average for the general population a as well. That is why $S_{\overline{x}}$ is known as a *standard error of the mean*. The last formula implies that *the larger the sample, the more accurate estimation of the mean and the lower its standard error are.* Moreover, the larger the variability of the original population, the larger the variability of the sample means, so the standard error of the mean increases along with the increase of the standard deviation of the population.

Distribution of sample means is always close to normal distribution, regardless of the population distribution from which the sample was taken. This is the main point of the statement also known as the *central limit theorem*. The following conclusions are the most important part of this theorem:

• sample means have approximately normal distribution, disregarding the distribution of original population from which they were taken;

• average value of all possible sample means equals to the average value within the population;

• average value of all possible average deviations in samples of the given size called standard error of the mean depends both on population standard deviation and sample size.

Increasing accuracy of estimates of the mean is reflected in the reduction of the standard error of the mean $S_{\overline{x}}$. Gathering a sufficient number of students, you can make a standard error of the mean arbitrarily small. In contrast to the standard deviation, the standard error of the mean says nothing about data scattering – it only shows the *accuracy* of sample estimate of the mean.

Even though the difference between standard deviation and standard error of the mean is quite obvious, they are frequently mixed up. Most researchers in their publications give value of the standard error of the mean which is clearly smaller than the standard deviation. They think that their data are more reliable in such a form. Maybe they are right. However, the standard error of the mean evaluates specifically accuracy in estimation of the mean, but not the data scattering which is in many cases more interesting than the error of the mean. As for standard deviation, it allows predetermining variability of the characteristic under study, and therefore helps the doctor to infer a conclusion from the analyses of a certain patient: are they within normal range or not. Therefore it is very important to know what exactly the author writes about – standard deviation or standard error of the mean.

2.3. INTERVAL ESTIMATES OF A RANDOM VARIABLE

Interval estimate of a random variable is a set of point estimates which covers an unknown parameter. Such interval is called *confidence interval* (Fig. 2.10). The lower boundary of the interval is the smallest value of the characteristic within the interval, and the upper boundary is the most important characteristic within it. The difference between upper and lower boundaries of the interval is actually the range of this interval.

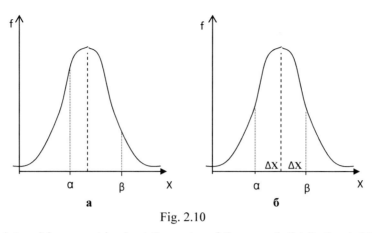

Fig. 2.10

If an interval is symmetric about the center of the normal distribution (with respect to mathematical expectation *a*), in such a way that both to the left and to the right intervals are equal Δx (Fig. 2.10.b), then the width of the interval will be $2\Delta x$. Sometimes half-width Δx is called confidence interval. The boundaries of the interval can be defined as α and β. Each confidence interval is associated to *confidence level P* or *reliability*. It helps to answer the question what is the probability that the unknown value of the estimated parameter of the population can be found within a given interval.

And though it cannot be shown precisely where the unknown parameter is on the number line, the confidence interval $2\Delta x$ within which the parameter is located with confidence probability *P*, can still be indicated.

LAPLACE'S FUNCTION

To solve the problem of the interval estimation it is necessary to pass from variable *x* to variable *t* in the Gaussian function. Suppose *(x – a)* is an actual deviation of the certain value of the random variable from mathematical expectation. Divide it by the standard deviation σ. The result of the division is represented as

$$t = \frac{x-a}{\sigma} = \frac{\Delta x}{\sigma}.$$

Thus, all values of the variable *x* are *normalized* or *standardized*. This parameter has the following meaning: it shows how many times the actual deviation is different from the standard. Therefore the parameter *t* is called the relative deviation. It is usually referred to as statistical criterion of the standard normal distribution. When testing statistical hypotheses its values allow either to accept or to reject proposed hypotheses.

Using the parameter *t*, the variable in the Gaussian function can be replaced

$$f(t) = \frac{1}{\sqrt{2\pi}} e^{-\frac{t^2}{2}}.$$

It makes the formula easier; and the diagram is shifted to the origin of coordinates, to the point with the coordinate $t = 0$ (with mathematical expectation equal to zero and $\sigma = 1$) with boundaries $-t$ and $+t$ (Fig. 2.11). Such diagram is more convenient to work with, since a great number of different random variables with normal distribution can be represented by repetitious diagram; and it gives an opportunity to create a universal algorithm for solving a variety of problems with different random variables. As it has been already mentioned above, the probability of values of the random variables to get into the given interval equals the area under the curve of the probability density function over this interval. Fig. 2.11 presents this shaded area. In mathematics, the area under the graph of a function is equal to the integral of this function. Then to

21

find the above mentioned probability within the interval from $-t$ to $+t$, the probability density function should be integrated into the given limits

$$P = S = \int_{-t}^{+t} f(t)dt.$$

Considering the symmetry of the interval, it is necessary to calculate the area from 0 to t and multiply it by two.

$$P = S = 2 \cdot \int_{0}^{+t} f(t)dt.$$

Substitute the Gaussian function into this formula.

$$P = S = 2 \cdot \int_{0}^{+t} \frac{1}{\sqrt{2\pi}} e^{-\frac{t^2}{2}} dt.$$

Values of this integral for different t were calculated by Pierre-Simon de Laplace. He presented them in a tabulated form. This table can be found in any mathematical handbook. Since values of this integral depend on the limit of t, the integral from the Gaussian function was named the Laplace's function and denoted as

$$\Phi(t) = \int_{0}^{+t} \frac{1}{\sqrt{2\pi}} e^{-\frac{t^2}{2}} dt.$$

Thus, the probability of the unknown value of the estimated parameter of the population to be found can be calculated using the formula: $P=2\Phi(t)$. If the interval is asymmetric

$$P = \Phi(t_2) - \Phi(t_1).$$

Note. Sometimes normal distribution tables instead of Laplace's function show the probability P itself or the significance level α; parameter t can be represented as z.

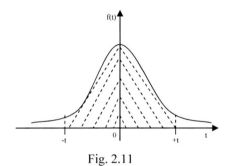

Fig. 2.11

CONFIDENCE INTERVAL FOR INDIVIDUAL VALUES OF STUDIED
CHARACTERISTIC WITH KNOWN GENERAL STANDARD DEVIATION

Suppose population X is distributed according to normal law $N(a,\sigma)$, where parameter σ is *known*. It is necessary to estimate confidence interval for the values of the characteristic under measurement. In this case, confidence interval formula can be derived from either formula $t = \frac{x-a}{\sigma}$ or $t = \frac{\Delta x}{\sigma}$. Half-width of the confidence interval equals

$$\Delta x = t \cdot \sigma \ .$$

Its center is at point a, left boundary is equal to $a - t\sigma$, right boundary equals $a + t\sigma$, and length of interval is equivalent to $2t\sigma$.

MEANING OF SIGMA, 2 SIGMA AND 3 SIGMA INTERVALS

The following formulas should be used to find probability of the normally distributed variable deviation from mathematical expectation on a certain value:

- for standard deviation, i.e. $\Delta x = \sigma$

$$P(|x - a| < \sigma) = 2\Phi(\frac{\sigma}{\sigma}) = 2\Phi(1) = 2 \cdot 0.3413 = 0.6826.$$

- for double standard deviation, i.e. $\Delta x = 2\sigma$

$$P(|x - a| < 2\sigma) = 2\Phi(\frac{2\sigma}{\sigma}) = 2\Phi(2) = 2 \cdot 0.4772 = 0.9544$$

- for triple standard deviation, i.e. $\Delta x = 3\sigma$

$$P(|x - a| < 3\sigma) = 2\Phi(\frac{3\sigma}{\sigma}) = 2\Phi(3) = 2 \cdot 0.49865 = 0.9973.$$

It may be concluded from these equations that in case of normal distribution, 68% of all values of a random variable are within the limits of standard deviation. If deviation is equal to two standard deviations, then within such interval boundaries lies approximately 95% of random variable values and less than 5% of them are left out. And finally, in case of interval with triple standard deviation 99% of all values lie within its boundaries, and only 1% of variable values are not included.

If the deviation is equal to two standard deviations, then approximately 95% of the values of a random variable is within this interval, and 5% of the values are at the tail. Finally, with 3 sigma interval, 99% of values are within it, and the tail gets only 1% of the values of the variable.

In medical practice confidence interval of individual values is usually defined as a sample mean plus or minus two standard deviations, which is really important when clarifying whether patient's analysis are within the "norm" boundaries or not. Practical application of σ in biological sciences is not limited only by morphological and anatomical studies. This figure works well in arranging ideas about seasonal changes in the nature, about distribution and dynamics in population of different organisms, as well as it helps in matters of selection and genetics.

Therefore, standard deviation is one of the most well-founded and effective descriptive statistics. However, if it is necessary to compare variability of the characteristics presented in different units of measurement (e.g. mm and gr.), it is impossible to use this figure, as it is measured in the same magnitude as the average quantity. In addition, the same standard deviation value (e.g. $\sigma = 2$) may point both to a very small ($\bar{x} = 100$) and a very large variability ($\bar{x} = 5$). To compare characteristics' variability in such cases it is better to use the *coefficient of variation*, which is equal to percentage ratio of the standard deviation to the arithmetic middling. It means that the coefficient of variation can be presented as a relative measure of dispersion, expressed as a percentage:

$$C_v = \frac{\sigma}{\bar{X}} \times 100\%$$

The smaller the coefficient of variation is, the more homogeneous sample is obtained. The variation is considered to be weak if it doesn't surpass 10%. If the coefficient of variation goes over $10 \div 20\%$, then the variation is called average. Strong variation happens when $C_v > 20\%$.

Statistical research has shown that the variability of the same characteristics expressed in terms of the coefficient of variation may vary both among different species and among different populations within the same species, and moreover these differences are often non-random and have a directed character. This was the reason to form unified methodological positions in the study of individual and evolutionary variation of organisms. The coefficient of variation between the different analyses and within the limits of one analysis evaluates *reproducibility* of a quantitative method. In other words, it reflects the degree of values identity received from repeating components in the sample. For example, consider the *reproducibility* of two methods of measuring the ESR. The first method (the modified Westergren method) gave the value of $\sigma = 1,0$ mm, where $\bar{x} = 10$ mm, and the second method (Linsenmayer method) - $\sigma = 15$ minutes and $\bar{x} = 180$ minutes.

The direct comparison of standard deviations gives no answer, since there are two values expressed in different units of measurement. Therefore, it is necessary to resort to the coefficient of variation: $V_1 = (1/10)*100 = 10\%; \quad V_2 = (15/180)*100 = 8,33\%$.

Conclusion: The reproducibility of the first validated method is lower ($10\% > 8,33\%$).

The coefficient of variation is not only used for comparative assessment of variation, but also to characterize the homogeneity of the population. The population is considered to be homogeneous, if the coefficient of variation does not exceed 33% (for the distributions that are close to normal).

INTERVAL ESTIMATES WITH T–DISTRIBUTION AND UNKNOWN GENERAL STANDARD DEVIATION

Development of the small sample theory was initiated by English statistician W.S. Gosset (whose works were printed under the pseudonym Student) in 1908. He proved that within a small sample there is a special distribution law. While assessing the results of a small sample, the size of the population variance should not be used in the calculations. To define the errors' possible limits the so-called t-distribution quantile should be used. According to the t-distribution, confidence interval depends both on confidence level P and on the sample size n. The smaller the sample size is, the more random, and therefore less reliable, the unknown parameter is within the interval.

The distribution of such samples is described with the W.S. Gosset's formula:

$$f(t_k) = \frac{\Gamma\left(\dfrac{k+1}{2}\right)}{\Gamma\left(\dfrac{k}{2}\right)\sqrt{\pi k}}\left(1+\frac{t^2}{k}\right)^{-\frac{k+1}{2}}$$

The letter Γ denotes the gamma function, the values of which, as it can be seen, depends on t and k. The k parameter is called the number of degrees of freedom. This value is not very different from the number of trials n. For different tasks $k = n - 1$, $k = n - 2$, $k = 2(n - 1)$. With increase of $k \to \infty$, which means that the number of trials $n \to \infty$ also increases, the values of the Gosset's function become closer to the Gaussian function, and t-distribution graph tends to take the form of a normal distribution graph. For small values of experiments Student's diagram is slanting and "blurred". This can be explained by the fact that at one and the same value of t, but different n, the probability will differ. Since the probability is numerically equal to the area of the curvilinear trapezoid, the height of the graphs will be different for different t. However, the total area under any trapezoid is the same, since the probability of being within an interval from $-\infty$ to $+\infty$ in any case equals 1 (or 100%).

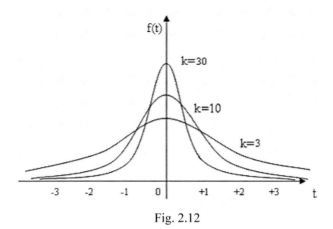

Fig. 2.12

The values of parameter t for different n; and different confidence levels P (or significance levels α) are summarized in the table for small samples. The table is called the Student table. The table shows that with the reduction of experiments number, but with the same confidence level, the parameter t increases, due to the need to extend the interval, so that it covered the unknown value of a random variable. On the other hand, with the same number of trials n, but with the increase of probability that the interval will cover the value of a random variable, it should be expanded, so the values of t increase.

In this case, attention can be drawn to the fact that with a high probability and with decreasing of the sample, t values rise more rapidly than at low probabilities, thus the interval will expand sharply. Due to last two circumstances the Student's parameter can be represented as $t_{p,k.}$

Note. *With a sufficiently large sample size, on the line denoted in the Student table by infinity symbol (∞), the parameter $t_{p,k}$ values are the same as the values of t from the Laplace table with the same probability.*

EXAMPLES

Variant 1
Suppose it is necessary to find the interval estimate for the mathematical expectation *a* with a *given confidence level* for a normally distributed population X in the case where the *population variance D is unknown*, and the sample is small. In other words, it is a problem of how precisely mathematical expectation can be estimated using the sample mean, how they differ from each other $\Delta x = (\bar{x} - a)$. Solution algorithm is as follows:

- it is necessary to find $\bar{x}$;
- to choose $t_{p,k,}$ in the Student table, knowing the degree of freedom $k = n - 1$ and confidence level P;
- using the sample calculate the standard deviation S_x or standard error $S_{\bar{x}}$;
- to evaluate the half-width of the confidence interval using the following formula

$$\Delta x = \frac{t_{p,k} \cdot S_x}{\sqrt{n}}$$

or $\Delta x = t_{pk} S_{\bar{x}}$;

- to estimate the confidence interval boundaries: $\alpha = \bar{x} - \Delta x$, $\beta = \bar{x} + \Delta x$.

Thus, the t-distribution quantile allows to find *the limiting random error* of the mathematical expectation evaluation with the given confidence level (or significance level), knowing the standard error for the sample data and the coefficient of $t_{p,k.}$

25

Variant 2

Suppose it is necessary *to find confidence probability P* of the fact that the *given confidence interval* (its half-width) Δx; covers mathematical expectation; the value of σ is unknown.

- to find $\bar{x}$ and S_x or $S_{\bar{x}}$;
- using the known value of Δx estimate parameter $t_{p,k}$ by formula:

$$t_{p,k} = \frac{\Delta x \sqrt{n}}{S_x};$$

$$\text{or } t_{p,k} = \frac{\Delta x}{S_{\bar{x}}};$$

- to calculate the degree of freedom $k = n - 1$;
- to find confidence probability (or significance level) in the Student table (*Appendix 2*), choosing the one that is equal or *the nearest lesser value $t_{p,k}$* in the table on the k line. The value of the confidence probability *P* or significance level α is indicated at the top of the column.

ONCE AGAIN ABOUT THE "MEASUREMENT ERROR" AND ITS EVALUATION

In conclusion, it is essential to repeat that the algorithm for calculating the errors in a small sample does not differ much from the similar calculations in a large sample. The difference is that the probability of the assertion for a small sample is somewhat smaller than for a large sample. In many cases, the discrepancy between the found boundaries can be quite significant; that hardly meets the needs of researchers. Therefore, a small sample should be used in a statistical study of medical events very carefully with appropriate theoretical and practical substantiation.

The standard error of the sample gives an idea of the non-sampling error, i.e. error with which the sample mean is the actual value of the general average. It shows what the error will be on the average, if from one and the same population a lot of samples of the same size are made. However, in each sample an error may differ significantly from the standard error. I.e. there is no guarantee that an error which was really made in the specific sampling study does not exceed the average error.

Therefore, it would be far more useful to know the boundaries within which a true error "almost certainly" is found in this particular sample. These boundaries (limits) are called *the limiting error of a sample* (is denoted by Δx). Limiting error of a sample indicates the limit, which is almost certainly not exceeded by the true error. In other words, the limiting error Δx shows the mistake which was really made with excess (possibly very notable) and thus ensures that the true error does not exceed Δx.

It can be said that measurement error will be the difference between the sample mean $\bar{x}$ and the mathematical expectation *a* (true mean or average in the population). The difference between them $\Delta x = |a - \bar{x}|$ is an error of measurement of the true mean. The value of such interval Δx is calculated by the following formula $\Delta x = t_{pk} S_{\bar{x}}$. Thus to find the limiting error of measurement with a given reliability (or confidence probability) the standard error must be multiplied by the quantile of Student. The quantile of Student can be found not only in the table, but also with the help of *Probability calculator* of the Statistica software package.

The limiting error formula can be presented the following way:

$$|a - \bar{x}| = t_{p,k} \cdot S_{\bar{x}}$$

From here it follows that:

$$a = \bar{x} \pm t_{p,k} \cdot S_{\bar{x}}$$

For example, finding the true value of a random variable "weight of a person" due to the sample data is written as

$$a = 72.6 \pm 1.2 \; (kg) \quad \text{with confidence probability equals to 95 \%.}$$

While calculating the error, quantity $t_{p,k}$ depends on the given confidence probability. In biology and medicine a rather high confidence probability is usually used: 95%, 99% and 99.9%.

If during the assessment of characteristic's variability it was said that 68% of the random variables are covered by σ–m interval, approximately 95% are covered with 2σ-m interval, and almost 99.8% are covered by 3σ–m interval, then in this case, it can be claimed that when the standard error is twice exceeded, the confidence interval will cover the random variable mathematical expectation with a probability of 95%; and when standard error is thrice exceeded, the confidence interval covers mathematical expectation (the true value) with 99.8% reliability.

From the analysis of the Student table and the given examples, an important conclusion can be drawn: if there have been few experiments n, there can be no hoping for a high reliability of the experiment results.

Nowadays, a small sample is used more widely than ever before. This method is used in the study of market structures, in selective inspection of products quality, in scientific research, medical examinations and in some other cases.

2.4. DISTRIBUTION DEVIATED FROM NORMAL; ITS NUMERICAL CHARACTERISTICS

When the distribution of the characteristic under study is not symmetrical around the mean and there are outlying cases in the sample, then distribution of this characteristic must be described using the median and percentiles. The basic concepts on which the decision on whether the distribution is normal or not, and the numerical characteristics of an asymmetric distribution of random variable are following:

Skewness:

$$A = \frac{\frac{1}{n} \cdot \sum_{i=1}^{n} (x_i - \bar{x})^3}{\frac{1}{n} \cdot \left[\sum_{i=1}^{n} (x_i - \bar{x})^2 \right]^{\frac{3}{2}}}$$

The skewness coefficient is a dimensionless value and is equal to zero at the symmetric distributions. If the distribution has a long part on the right off the nod, then the skewness is called positive, and the distribution with a long part of the frequency curve to the left from the nod, is called negative skewness.

Kurtosis:

$$E = \frac{\frac{1}{n} \cdot \sum_{i=1}^{n} (x_i - \bar{x})^4}{\frac{1}{n} \cdot \left[\sum_{i=1}^{n} (x_i - \bar{x})^2 \right]^{2}} - 3$$

Kurtosis coefficient quantifies the distribution peakedness. For normal distribution it equals zero. The distribution with the curves that are peaked has a leptokurtosis, and with flat-topped curves – a platykurtosis.

The distribution can be considered to be normal, if the values of these parameters are close to zero (less than 0.5). Also, they are compared to their own mistakes. Skewness and kurtosis should not exceed their non-sampling error more than three times. I.e. they should be of the same magnitude. Under this condition the distribution can be considered to be normal.

Quartiles − are 3 points of the characteristic value, which divide the ordered (ascending) set of observations into 4 equal in size parts. First quartile corresponds to the 25th percentile, the second – to the 50th percentile, or median, the third quartile corresponds to the 75th percentile.

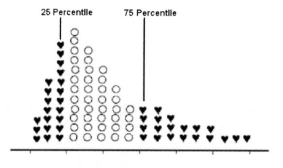

Fig. 2.13

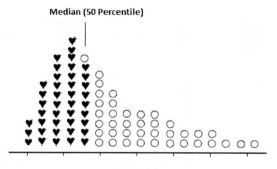

Fig. 2.14

Maximum – is the largest value in the sample.

Median – is a value of the characteristic, which divides ordered (ranged) set of data in half so that one part of all values appears to be less than median, and the other part – larger. This is the second quartile (Fig. 2.13 and 2.14).

Minimum – is the smallest value in the sample.

Mode – is the only *location parameter* for the description of nominal qualitative characteristics. (*Mo*) – is such a numerical value, which is most frequently found in the sample. Mode, or characteristic modal interval, corresponds to the highest rise (peak) of the frequency distribution graph. Mode can also be calculated for qualitative ordinal characteristics.

Percentiles – are 99 points – values of the characteristic. They divide ordered (ascending) set of observations into 100 parts that are equal in size. In other words, the first quartile – is the 25th percentile, the second quartile – is the 50th percentile, and the third quartile – is the 75th percentile.

Range (dispersion) – is the difference between the maximum and the minimum values of a certain ordered sample. The more characteristic under measurement varies, the larger the range is, and vice versa.

Box & Whisker Plot – is a graphical representation of the asymmetrically distributed values. They look as follows:

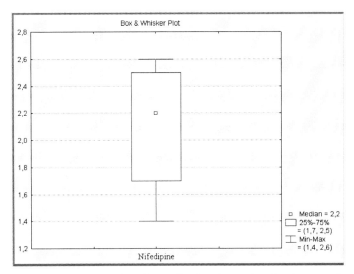

Variants of the variable's value (V) shown in the chart when having certain percentiles (quartiles) can be written as follows:

The median values $V_{0,5} = 1,3$ (sometimes is written as $Me = 2.2$; the value of the 25th percentile $V_{0,25} = 1.7$; the value of the 75th percentile $V_{0,75} = 2.5$.

Median confidence interval algorithm

1. It is necessary to rank the values of the characteristic under study in ascending order. To do this, in the package Statistica choose **Variables** and **Rank** in ascending order.

2. For samples of the size $n>50$ confidence interval is expressed by the following formula:

$$x_k \leq Me \leq x_{k-n+1,}$$

where

$$k = \frac{1}{2} \cdot \left(n - 1{,}64 \cdot \sqrt{n} - 1\right), \text{ where } \alpha = 0.1;$$

$$k = \frac{1}{2} \cdot \left(n - 1{,}96 \cdot \sqrt{n} - 1\right), \text{ where } \alpha = 0.05;$$

$$k = \frac{1}{2} \cdot \left(n - 2{,}58 \cdot \sqrt{n} - 1\right), \text{ where } \alpha = 0.01.$$

3. For values of $n \leq 50$ refer to the table in **Appendix 5.** The tables indicates the numbers of order statistics, which contain the median for $\alpha = 0.1$, $\alpha = 0.05$ and $\alpha = 0.01$.

Confidence interval for relative frequency

Interval estimation is quite challenging when calculating a proportion. It is denoted by

$$p_d = \frac{m}{n}.$$

Finding the error in calculation of the proportion is the task of interval estimation of the proportion in the population $p_{ген}$ using the proportion found in the sample p_d. There are several ways to solve this problem. By analogy with the confidence interval for the mathematical expectation write a formula for the error in the measurement of a true proportion:

$$p_{d\lim it} = p_d \pm t\overline{S}_{p_d} .$$

Then the boundaries for proportion's true value are calculated by the following formula:

$$p_d \pm t\left(\sqrt{\frac{p_d(1-p_d)}{n}}\right)$$

In case of a large sample with a significance point **p** = 0.05, the value $t = 1.96$.

In case of a small sample **Student's t-quantile** can be used, but only taking into account the degree of freedom and significance point in the Student table, or indicating them in the **Probability calculator** while working with the Statistica package.

However, to use **Student's t-quantile** it is essential to simultaneously perform the following conditions:

$np_d \geq 5$;
$n(1-p_d) \geq 5$;
$0.3 \leq p_d \leq 0.7$,

n – sample size, p_d – relative frequency.

In small samples more complex formulas are used, if the conditions of t appliance are not fulfilled. This difficulty can be gone around by using **Appendix 6** or alignment chart 95% of confidence intervals for the proportions, calculated on the basis of the binomial distribution (Fig. 2.15).

When the sample size or the observed proportion are very small and thus normal distribution cannot be used, it is necessary to use *binomial distribution*, which with the increasing of the sample size comes closer to the normal distribution. It is extremely important in medical research where samples of a small size and rather rare events can often occur.

If, for instance, when testing a new drug within a small sample, it has not shown the side effects, then the sample estimate of the side effect risk proportion equals zero, and therefore, the confidence interval is equal to zero. But this does not mean that the drug is safe!

To determine the confidence interval for the binomial distribution, it is necessary to find the point on the nomogram (Fig. 2.15) horizontal axis that corresponds to the sample rate p_d. After that it is required to draw a perpendicular exactly from this point and see where this line is intersected by a couple of curves marked with a number which equals sample size. Vertical coordinates of the intersection points will be the boundaries of the 95% confidence interval. Assume that $p_d = 0$ and sample size equals 50, then lower boundary is equal to zero and upper boundary is equal to about 0.1. It means that with a probability of 95% it can be claimed that the risk of side effects will not exceed 10%. Note that the interval becomes wider with the reduction in sample size. Thus, if the sample size was 10, the risk of side effects would not exceed 33%.

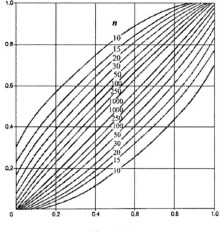

Fig. 2.15

2.5. DETERMINATION OF REQUIRED SAMPLE SIZE

DETERMINATION OF THE SAMPLE SIZE OF QUANTITATIVE CHARACTERISTIC

From the error formula the number of units (or sample size) n is calculated using the following formula:

$$n = \frac{t^2 S^2}{\Delta x^2}$$

For reliability of 95% t value is 2, S – standard deviation of the characteristic in the population (or sample), Δx – accuracy of the result, or the maximum allowable difference between the sample mean and population mean.

One of the sampling method problems is that unless the selection is made, the value of S in the formula for the sample size is not known, so for the final sampling it is necessary to do a trial or model sampling to determine S. This value for the population can be taken from the literature or the initial phase of the research.

DETERMINATION OF THE SAMPLE SIZE TO ESTIMATE THE PROPORTION OF QUALITATIVE CHARACTERISTIC

The formula for calculating the sample size to determine the unknown value of the qualitative characteristic proportion in the population with a given confidence level can be derived using the standard error formula for a qualitative characteristic in the sample. This formula is:

$$n = \frac{t^2 p_d (1 - p_d)}{\Delta p_d^{\,2}}$$

Where Δp_d – accuracy of the result, or the maximum allowable difference between the sample proportion and the proportion in the population. Parameter t for the confidence level of 95% equals 2.

To determine the required size of the ***two samples***, Altman's nomogram can be used (***Appendix* 7).**

The necessary conditions for its use are following:
- statistical power is set at the level of 80% – 90% (0.8 – 0.9);
- statistical significance of differences must not exceed 0.05;
- it is essential to determine the minimal standardized difference of the parameter under study in compared groups.

For *quantitative measurements in independent groups* standardized difference is equal to Δ / S, and in *dependent groups* $2\Delta / S$. Δ – *is the absolute value of the minimum mean difference with clinical significance.* And S – is a priori known from previous studies standard deviation of the characteristic in this category of experimental units.

Standardized difference *for binary (qualitative) characteristic* is evaluated by the following formula:

$$\frac{P_{d1} - P_{d2}}{\sqrt{\dfrac{P_{d1} + P_{d2}}{2} \left(1 - \dfrac{P_{d1} + P_{d2}}{2}\right)}}$$

P_{d1} and P_{d2} – are the proportions in each sample.

Values of sample size for independent samples must be divided by 2, if they are identical. If the sizes are not the same, then the value is calculated with the formula $N_1 = N(1+k)^2/4k$, where N – sample size derived from the nomogram, the ratio of sample sizes $k = n_1/n_2$, and samples sizes themselves: $n_1 = N_1/(1+k)$, $n_2 = kN_1/(1+k)$.

31

Standardized deviation is found on the left axis of the nomogram. This point is connected to the point on the axis of power at the right side of the nomogram. The required sample size is at the point where the drawn line intersects with the axis of size (middle axis).

CHAPTER 3

FUNDAMENTALS OF THE THEORY OF HYPOTHESES

3.1. NOTION OF HYPOTHESIS. THE TYPES OF HYPOTHESES. DECISION CRITERIA

The word hypothesis comes from Greek meaning a "supposition". Solution of statistical problems usually implies two stages: a supposition about the distribution of a random variable in question and the study of this variable in the context of the supposition put forward. If the sampling data is known but the law of the distribution of the general population is unknown, there are grounds to suppose that the law takes a particular form. For instance, the following hypothesis is set forth: **the general population is distributed according to the normal law**. Hence, it's the hypothesis on a type of the presupposed distribution.

There are cases when the distribution law is known meanwhile its parameters are unknown. Consequently, if it is correct to say that the unknown parameter σ is equal to the defined value σ_0, the hypothesis that $\sigma = \sigma_0$ is put forward. This is the hypothesis on the presupposed parameter value of the known distribution.

Other hypotheses are also possible: on the equality of parameters of two populations or more, on the independence of samples, on the accuracy (or absence) of differences between sampling arithmetic means or variances (see variance analysis).

A hypothesis can be correct or incorrect, that is why it is necessary to test it. Since this test is carried out using statistical methods, it is called statistical. Thus, a hypothesis on a type of the unknown distribution or on its parameters is referred to as **statistical hypothesis**.

Along with the hypothesis H_0 an alternative to it hypothesis H_1 is examined. If the first hypothesis is rejected, the alternative one comes into effect. It is necessary to distinguish these two hypotheses.

For example, the null hypothesis H_0 is the following: statistical expectation of the general population is equal to 1 ($a = 1$).

The alternative hypothesis H_1 is $a>1$, or $a<1$, or $a1 \neq a2$.

As a result of the statistical test of the hypotheses, an incorrect decision might be made, i.e. some errors might be committed. The error of the first kind (Type I error) is the incorrect rejection of a null hypothesis and the false acceptance of the alternative one. The probability of making type I error is usually denoted by α, as this takes place $\alpha = P(H_1/H_0)$ means the probability to accept H_1 if the hypothesis H_0 is true. For instance, while analyzing the differences between two groups, the value of α will reflect the percentage of cases when nonexistent differences are found. To simplify it is possible to say that α is the probability of the null hypothesis validity.

The type I error is called the *level of significance*. The statistical significance of the result is an estimated measure of the confidence in its "validity".

The significance level is mostly (especially in medicine) equaled to 0.05 or 0.01. If, for example, the significance level is equal to 0.05, it means that 5 times in 100 cases we risk to commit the type I error (to reject the null hypothesis). This is the reason why this level is sometimes called the level of the risk or the probability of making the type I error that is connected with the appliance of the result to the whole population. In many statistical software packages the designation *p* or *p-level (value)* is used instead of α. This indicator is in descending correspondence with the reliability of the result $\alpha = 1$ -confidence figure. The higher *p-level p-value* corresponds to the lower level of the confidence.

In medical research if the probability of the null hypothesis is less than 0.05, it is rejected; if the probability of the null hypothesis is more than 0.05, it is accepted.

The error of the second type (Type II error) means the probability of the acceptance of H_0 if the hypothesis H_1 is true. It is presented as $\text{ß} = P(H_0/H_1)$.

It is necessary to emphasize that the significance level 0.05 is optimal to detect critical value of statistical criteria. In the above-mentioned hypothesis on differences when α is 0.01, false conclusions on the existence of differences are likely to be made. The probability of making a false conclusion goes down to 1%; meanwhile, the probability of finding differences where they are no differences goes up.

The probability of the incorrect rejection of a true null hypothesis and the acceptance of an alternative hypothesis instead varies from case to case. It is clear that the quantity of significant (at the chosen level) results discovered by accident depends on the quantity of analyses carried out on the basis of the population data. Some statistical methods, including many comparisons and as a consequence, repeating this type of errors, demands special correction or adjustment to the total number of comparisons. However, many statistical methods (especially simple methods of exploratory data analysis do not suggest any approaches to solve the problem. That is why the researcher has to be careful in estimation of reliability of unexpected results.

The statistical test is a random variable that helps to make a decision whether to accept or reject the H_0 hypothesis.

The statistical test is a random variable that helps to make a decision whether to accept or reject the H_0 hypothesis. In other words, it is a rigid mathematical rule according to which a statistical hypothesis is accepted or rejected. Each criterion is formed differently depending on the type of the hypothesis.

The group of statistical tests that is reckoned with the parameters of the normal distribution of a characteristic (means or variance) is called parametric. These tests are used to rapidly estimate reliability of differences in control and experimental groups or to establish the connection between variables. Examples of the parametric criteria:

- $t_{p,k}$ – Student's t test;
- F – Fisher's test (Fisher Ronald Aylmer).

Nonparametric tests do not demand the normal distribution of the characteristic. They are based on operating on statistical frequency and ranks. Rank of the variable is its number in the rank-order. Such nonparametric tests as Kolmogorov-Smirnov test, Wilcoxon test, Mann-Withney test, Friedman test, Spearman test, χ^2 Person test etc are widely applied. They are also used to estimate rapidly reliability of differences in control and experimental groups or to establish the connection between variables.

NB. *If the normal distribution is observed, parametric tests contribute to a quick response. But if the condition is not completely fulfilled, it's quick response capability decreases dramatically, and the probability to detect differences with the help of nonparametric tests increases.*

Concordance test is a statistical test destined for finding discrepancy between statistical model and real data described by it. These tests are applied when identifying the degree of compliance between random variables distribution and experimental data.

Critical region is the population value of the test whereby the null hypothesis is rejected.

Null hypothesis acceptance region (tolerance region) is the population value of the test whereby the null hypothesis is accepted.

If the significance level is equal to 0.05 (confidence figure is equal to 0.95), the critical value -1.96 corresponds to the left border, and the critical value +1.96 corresponds to the right border (see the table of the Laplace function, *Appendix* 1)

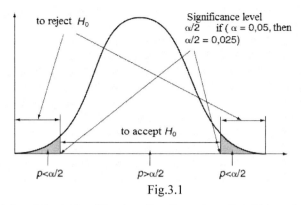

Fig.3.1

The Fig.3.1 and the table of Laplace functions show that if the value, calculated with the t-test formula when the significance value equals to 0.05, falls within the interval from -1.96 to +1.96, the null hypothesis is accepted, otherwise it is rejected. They also show that the false null hypothesis acceptance region is divided into two parts (distribution tail area more than +1.96 and less than -1.96). Both parts of a critical region are used when the hypothesis is not explicit. For example, when studying the influence of a low-salt diet on arterial tension (AT), we cannot suppose that the diet only reduces it. It is very likely that there will be cases when the patient's AT will be raised. I.e. decrease or increase of AT is not irregular. To test such hypotheses **two-tailed tests** are used. One-sided hypothesis and one-sided test are used when the researcher is convinced that the results will be only explicit. For example, when the purpose is to define how alcohol affects the ability to drive a car, it is difficult to expect that the alcohol will improve driving skills; that is why one-sided test is used. For instance, distributions inequality of two populations ($\sigma_x^2 > \sigma_y^2$) is tested by one-sided Fisher's exact test.

Note. In the Student's t-test critical points for two-sided tests are marked, consequently if the significance value is 0.01, we should look for a critical point for one-sided test in the Student's t-test table for a value that is two times bigger, i.e. for 0.02. If computer software calculates the significance value for one-sided test, it is necessary to multiple it by two when we are interested in two-sided test!!

*Note. Quite often such parameter as **strength of test** is used to estimate the results of the research. If β is the probability of the error of the second kind, then **the strength of test is 1 - β**. It means that the critical region should be formed according to the chosen significance value so that the strength of the test would be maximal.*

Algorithm of statistic hypothesis testing

1. To formulate a null hypothesis H_0 and its rival hypothesis H_1 disposing sampling data ($x_1, x_2, ..., x_n$);

2. To assign the significance value (α =0.1; 0.01; 0.05; 0.001);

3. To choose one of the above-mentioned tests depending on the hypothesis, the type of measurement, the type of variables etc.

4. To calculate the value of a statistical test using random data ($x_1, x_2, ..., x_n$) and compare it with the critical value of the test taken from relevant tables. If the value of the calculated test is more than the critical table value ($t_{cal.} > t_{crit.}$), then H_0 is rejected, and H_1 hypothesis is accepted; if not, the H_0 hypothesis is accepted, and it is considered that H_0 is not in contrast with random data (in this case the probability of the error is equal to α).

The degree of freedom of the parameter is defined with the number of experiments, according to which this parameter is calculated deducting the number of invariables found in the result of these experiments independent one from another. For example, when the confidence interval, covering the statistical expectation, is defined, the number of experiments is equal to n, the degree of freedom is $k = n - 1$, as long as the number of invariables is equal to 1. If the pur-

35

pose is to find the connection between two variables, the formula is $k = n - 2$ since the number of invariables is equal to 2.

HYPOTHESIS TESTING ON THE EQUALITY OF MATHEMATICAL EXPECTATIONS OF TWO NORMAL DISTRIBUTIONS WITH UNKNOWNS BUT EQUAL DISTRIBUTIONS

Suppose $x_1,...,x_{n1}$ and $y_1,...,y_{n2}$ are two independent samples from normally distributed relevant general populations X and Y, sample numbers are n_1 and n_2. The principle of the null hypothesis H_0 is that the difference between mean values is irregular, that means that the average populations equal to each other ($a_1 = a_2$). The principle of the alternative hypothesis H_1 is that statistical expectations are not equal to each other ($a_1 \neq a_2$). Sample numbers n_1 and n_2 are relevant. Let us form a test for testing this hypothesis basing on the following idea: since the approximate image of mathematical expectation is defined with a random mean, the comparison of these two random means $\bar{x}$ и $\bar{y}$ is to be taken as the basis. If two variables are distributed normally, their common difference $(\bar{x} - \bar{y})$ will be normally distributed (if the null hypothesis H_0 on the equality of average populations is true).

The test of a hypothesis on equality of mathematical expectations of two populations has significant practical importance. Effectively, sometimes the mean $\bar{x}$ of one set of observations differs from the mean of $\bar{y}$ of another set. The question now arises of whether this difference can be explained by a random error in experiments or it is not random. In other words, whether experiment outcomes are samples of two populations with common mean values.

Let us show the intervals of the range of values of a variable in one or another sample for two cases.

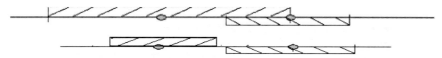

Fig. 3.2

Fig. 3.2 shows that the mean values for two cases are common, so their difference is common, but the range of values in the first case is bigger than in the second one. Since values of a random variable in samples in the first case are overlapped, the difference of their means (as well as their average populations) in the second case is more reliable than in the first one. Hence, it is necessary to compare the difference of the means with the range of differences, or to be more exact, with a standard error of the mean difference. If the mean difference is greater than this error, it will be a rough estimate of the differences in the mean values.

If the number of objects in two groups is common, this range of difference is to be counted using the following formula:

$$S_\Delta = \sqrt{\frac{(n_x - 1)S_x^2 + (n_y - 1)S_y^2}{n_x + n_y - 2}}$$

Subsequently, the standard error of the mean differences is

$$\bar{S}_\Delta = S_\Delta \cdot \sqrt{\frac{1}{n_x} + \frac{1}{n_y}}$$

After the division of the absolute mean differences by the standard error, the test formula will be

$$T = \frac{|\overline{X} - \overline{Y}|}{\sqrt{(n_1 - 1) \cdot S_x^2 + (n_2 - 1) \cdot S_y^2}} \cdot \sqrt{\frac{n_1 \cdot n_2 (n_1 + n_2 - 2)}{n_1 + n_2}}.$$

The T variable has the Student's distribution c $k = n_1 + n_2 - 2$ degrees of freedom. Let us define the significance value α and test the null hypothesis. The critical parameter $t_{p,k}$ is found in the Student's table. If $T \geq t_{\text{crit.}}$, the null hypothesis is rejected or vice versa.

Note 1. *If the number of objects in the groups in question is common, the test is calculated as follows*:

$$T = \frac{|\overline{X} - \overline{Y}|}{\sqrt{\frac{S_x^2}{n} + \frac{S_y^2}{n}}}$$

Note 2. *Before using the algorithm, it is necessary to test the hypothesis on distributions equality.*

3.2. HYPOTHESIS TESTING ON THE EQUALITY OF MATHEMATICAL EXPECTATIONS OF TWO NORMAL DISTRIBUTIONS.

HYPOTHESIS TESTING ON EQUALITY OF MATHEMATICAL EXPECTATIONS OF TWO NORMAL DISTRIBUTIONS WITH UNKNOWNS AND UNEQUAL DISTRIBUTIONS

Let us formulate the statistical hypotheses. The null hypothesis H_0 consists in the fact that the difference of means is not random, subsequently, its average populations are common ($a_1 = a_2$). The alternative hypothesis H_1 consists in the fact that statistical expectations are not common ($a_1 \neq a_2$). Sample numbers are n_1 and n_2. The criterion of testing of this hypothesis is the following:

$$T = \frac{|\overline{X} - \overline{Y}|}{\sqrt{\frac{S_x^2}{n_1} + \frac{S_y^2}{n_2}}}$$

In this case the number of degrees of freedom is calculated with a complicated formula:

$$k = \frac{(n_1 - 1) \cdot (n_2 - 1) \cdot \left(\frac{S_x^2}{n_1} + \frac{S_y^2}{n_2} \right)^2}{(n_2 - 1) \cdot \left(\frac{S_x^2}{n_1} \right)^2 + (n_1 - 1) \left(\frac{S_y^2}{n_2} \right)^2}$$

However, computer statistical data-processing operation allows fast and simple calculation of all variants of tests. If we take the significance level α and start testing the null hypothesis, we will have to find the critical value $t_{p,k}$ in the Student's table. If $T \geq t_{\text{crit}}$, we reject the null hypothesis or vice versa.

Note. *Before using this algorithm, it is necessary to test the hypothesis on the distribution equality.*

HYPOTHESIS TESTING ON THE VARIANCES EQUALITY OF TWO NORMAL DISTRIBUTIONS

In the previous paragraph when testing the hypothesis on equation of mathematical expectations, it was guessed that distributions of these populations are common. How to prove it if only sampling distributions values are known? The objective of testing the hypothesis on the distributions equality has self-contained interest. Since the distribution characterizes the accuracy of an indicator or a technological process, after proving the distributions inequality, it is possible to talk about the accuracy of an indicator or a technological process.

Let us assume that X and Y are two random variables that have normal distributions and unknown distributions σ_x^2 and σ_y^2.

Independent samples with the following parameters n_1, S_x^2, n_2, S_y^2 are taken from these populations. It is required to test the null hypothesis H_0: $\sigma_x^2 = \sigma_y^2$ when the alternative one-sided (directional) hypothesis is H_1: $\sigma_x^2 > \sigma_y^2$ on the condition that the significance level is α. Starting sample estimations, as F criterion we use the dependency of the bigger sample distribution to the smaller one. This random variable F has F-Fisher's distribution with the following numbers of the degrees of freedom $k_1 = n_1 - 1$ and $k_2 = n_2 - 1$, where k_1 is the number of that sample whose sample distribution turned out to be bigger. In Fisher's table there is a number k_2. The critical value $F_{crit.}$ is at the intersection of the raw and the column.

$$F = \frac{S_{max}^2}{S_{min}^2}$$

Apparently, if the distributions are equal, F-criteria is 1. If it is bigger than one, it is necessary to reject the null hypothesis. The question arises what is the value of F needs to be so that the H_0 would be rejected, in other words, what are the critical values of the criterion? Again everything depends on the significance value that was chosen and the number of sampling experiments. To test the null hypothesis, it is necessary to compare the result of Fisher's test $F_{calc.}$ with the critical value $F_{p,k}$ from the Fisher's distributions tables. If $F_{calc.} \geq F_{crit.}$, the null hypothesis is to be rejected. Since the $F_{crit.}$ value depends on three variables: the significance value α and two degrees of freedom k_1 и k_2, those three-dimensional tables are composed for all values of α (**Appendix 4**).

CONFIDENCE INTERVAL CONSTRUCTION FOR THE MEAN DIFFERENCE

Limits of the confidence interval for the mean difference are calculated with the formula $\Delta \pm t \cdot \bar{S}_\Delta$ where the variable $\bar{S}_\Delta$ is the standard error of the mean differences. It consists of standard errors for x and y. If the sample numbers are equal to each other $\bar{S}_\Delta = \sqrt{\bar{S}_x^2 + \bar{S}_y^2}$; if not,

$$\bar{S}_\Delta = S_\Delta \cdot \sqrt{\frac{1}{n_x} + \frac{1}{n_y}}$$

Quantile of Student's t-distribution for the 95% of the interval is approximately equal to 1.96 in case of a large sample ($n = \infty$). For other cases it is to be found in the Student's table for the degree of freedom $n_1 + n_2 - 2$. It is possible to use **the Probability Calculator** in the statistical software package STATISTICA.

If the confidence interval does not include zero, an alternative hypothesis on the existence of differences with the known significance value should be accepted.

METHOD OF REPEATING TESTS

In medicine the method of repeating tests is associated with the method of comparison of population means, but is significantly more sensitive. Earlier in order to estimate the efficiency of treatment, it was necessary to chose two groups. The members of one of them were treated; meanwhile, the members of another one were not. Now we choose one group that is tested twice. The value of the characteristic of the illness of each patient is estimated before and after the treatment. Such samples are called dependent. In such a case the characteristic should be normally distributed, as well as its value difference.

One of standard medical tasks where the method of repeating tests can be applied is to know whether a medicine has an effect or not. In such experiments it is usually important to exclude psychotherapeutic influence. That is why the essence of the experiment is in the fact that in one of the experiments its participants take placebo, which is ineffective; and in another one they take the medicine being studied. The participants do not know what they take in both cases.

In case of using one sample in the experiment, each object under observation gives two values of the random variable x_i and x_i' in two experiments (pair of values). In this case x_i is the value of the random variable for i-th object before the experiment, x_i' is the value of this variable for the same object after the experiment.

The difference of these values (difference for only one object of observation) will be denoted as $d_i = x_i - x_i'$. This idea of solving the problem using repeating tests in one sample is the same as the comparison of two samples.

It is necessary to compare the mean difference with the error in finding of the mean difference. They can be compared also using the t-test (*paired* samples Student's *t*-test). It is formed as follows:

$$T = \frac{\overline{d}}{S_{\overline{d}}}$$

Thus, the problem solving algorithm is:

1. To put forward the null hypothesis H_0 on the absence of changes (the factor does not influence) and an alternative hypothesis H_1 on the presence of changes (the factor influences).

2. To calculate the variation value for each object $d_i = x_i - x_i'$

3. To calculate the mean value of these changes using the formula

$$\overline{d} = \frac{\sum d_i}{n} = \frac{\sum (x_i - x_i')}{n}$$

4. To calculate the standard error of the mean difference:

$$S_{\overline{d}} = \sqrt{\frac{\sum (d_i - \overline{d})^2}{n(n-1)}}$$

5. To calculate the value of the paired samples Student's *t*-test:

$$T = \frac{\overline{d}}{S_{\overline{d}}}$$

6. To detect the critical value of the paramater t_{pk} for the given significant value α for the number of degrees of freedom $k = n - 1$.

7. To compare the found value $T_{calc.}$ with $t_{crit.}$ from the table. If $T_{calc.} \geq t_{crit.}$, the null hypothesis on the absence of influence is rejected, and the alternative hypothesis on the influence

of the factor is accepted. Or, in other words, if the significance value $\alpha > 0.05$, the null hypothesis on the absence of differences before and after the interference. If $\alpha \leq 0.05$, an alternative hypothesis on the presence of differences with given level of significance is accepted.

Taking into account such comparisons, the question on the estimation of confidence interval for the mean difference arises. Limits of the interval can be calculated with the following formula:

$$\overline{d} \pm t \cdot S_{\overline{d}}$$

Quantile of Student's t-distribution for the 95% interval in case of a large sample is approximately equal to 1.96. For other cases it is to be found in the Student's table with the given degree of freedom. It is possible to use **Probability Calculator** in the statistical software package STATISTICA. If the confidence interval does not include zero, the alternative hypothesis on the existence of differences with the given significance value should be accepted.

Note. Rather often the mean values in connected groups do not differ. That is why the change is estimated relating to the initial level.

The results are presented as follows:

$$\frac{(\overline{X}_t - \overline{X}_0) \cdot 100\%}{\overline{X}_0}$$

If the value of the parameter is positive, the indicator is considered to be increased. If the value of the parameter is negative, the minus symbol is ignored, and the indicator decreases.

Very important note. Statistically significant differences should not be accepted as the ultimate truth. Sometimes the clinical importance turns out to be low even if the mean difference is statistically significant. Especially, it is easy to see it after confidence interval construction for the mean difference. Confidence intervals allow determining among statistically significant effects those that have clinical importance. If the clinical importance is found only due to the large sample but not the effect size, the interval will "find it out". If estimating the efficiency of antihypertensive medicine, arterial tension goes down by 5 units with the standard deviation decreasing by 10 units in each group of 100 people, the calculated criterion will exceed the critical value at the significance value equal to 0.05. However, the confidence interval for the mean difference will have the limits.

$$5 \pm 1{,}96 \cdot \sqrt{\frac{10^2}{100} + \frac{10^2}{100}} \quad, or \quad 5 \pm 2.77$$

As it can be seen, antihypertensive effect is not high, and its statistical value is defined by the large sample.

3.3. HYPOTHESIS TESTING ON THE EQUALITY OF FRACTIONS OF TWO BINOMINAL DISTRIBUTIONS

In medical science one often has to deal with qualitative characters, i.e. those object indicators that can be described with words. For example, who are males and females among the objects of the medical supervision, or the way the patients feel after surgery can be described as "good", "satisfactory", and "unsatisfactory".

Suppose in the group of patients of 60 people having had the ulcer of stomach treated in an old manner, 15 patients have complications. And in the group of 40 people who had it treated in a new manner, only 5 patients have complications. Then the fraction of those who have complications in the first group is $15/60 = 1/4$ or 25%, and in the second group it is $5/40 = 1/8$ or 12.5%.

Since we calculate fractions using a formula which is actually the statistical definition of probability, this fraction can be denoted by the same letter but with the indicator p_d in order to distinguish the fraction from the confidence probability P. The formula for the fractions p_d is the following:

$$p_d = \frac{m}{n}$$

The fractions calculated according to the sample are analogues of the arithmetic average. Every sampling fraction is the estimation of the population $\hat{p}_d$. Let us put the question forward what is the degree of reliability for the general population?

It is necessary to put forward the statistical hypotheses.

The null hypothesis H_0: fractions do not differ in the population,

The alternative hypothesis H_1: fractions differ in the population.

The standard error of the fraction has the formula which we present without a proof:

$$\overline{S}_{p_d} = \sqrt{\frac{p_d(1-p_d)}{n}}$$

Then the error of estimation of fractions differences will be calculated with the formula:

$$\overline{S}_{p_{1d}-p_{2d}} = \sqrt{\overline{S}^2_{p_{1d}} + \overline{S}^2_{p_{2d}}} \ .$$

Developing the test and using already known logic, let us compare the fractions difference with the error of estimation of the difference. As a result, we get the following:

$$T = \frac{sampling\_fractions\_difference}{standard\_error\_of\_the\_sampling\_fractions\_difference}$$

$$T = \frac{p_{1d} - p_{2d}}{\sqrt{\overline{S}^2_{p_{1d}} + \overline{S}^2_{p_{2d}}}}$$

Or:

$$T = \frac{(p_{1d} - p_{2d})}{\sqrt{\dfrac{p_{1d}(1-p_{1d})}{n_1} + \dfrac{p_{2d}(1-p_{2d})}{n_2}}}$$

If we combine observations from both samples while estimating the distribution, the sensitivity of Student's t-test will increase. To calculate a new parameter, let us consider that the sampling fractions $\hat{p}_{1d} = \dfrac{m_1}{n_1}$ and $\hat{p}_{2d} = \dfrac{m_2}{n_2}$ are two estimations of the same fraction $\hat{p}_d$ that we can estimate as follows:

$$p_d = \frac{m_1 + m_2}{n_1 + n_2}, \quad \text{then} \quad S_{p_d} = \sqrt{p_d(1-p_d)} \ .$$

This is how we get the standard error of fractions difference.

$$\overline{S}_{p_{1d}-p_{2d}} = \sqrt{\frac{S^2_{p_d}}{n_1} + \frac{S^2_{p_d}}{n_2}} = \sqrt{p_d(1-p_d) \cdot \left(\frac{1}{n_1} + \frac{1}{n_2} \right)}$$

41

Substituting the found estimation in the *t*-test formula, we get:

$$T = \frac{(p_{1d} - p_{2d})}{\sqrt{p_d(1-p_d)\cdot\left(\dfrac{1}{n_1}+\dfrac{1}{n_2}\right)}}$$

The algorithm of the hypotheses testing is analogical to the above-mentioned cases. It is necessary to compare the found value of T_{calc} with t_{crit} from the table. If $T_{calc} \geq t_{crit}$, the null hypothesis on the absence of influence is rejected, and the alternative one on influence of the factor is accepted. Or in other words, if the significance value while testing the null hypothesis is more than 0.05, the null hypothesis on the absence of difference of relative frequencies is accepted. If the significance value is less than 0.05, the alternative hypothesis on the existence of the difference of relative frequencies is accepted.

Note. *If the characteristic in question has been studied not in the whole group of objects of observation, but only at their part, then the number of patients whose characteristic has been studied but not the whole sample should be taken for 100%.*

Yates's correction for continuity

To compensate the redundant value of *T* because of the discreteness of its values the following correction is introduced:

$$T = \frac{\left|(p_{1d} - p_{2d})\right| - \dfrac{1}{2}(\dfrac{1}{n_1}+\dfrac{1}{n_2})}{\sqrt{p_d(1-p_d)\cdot\left(\dfrac{1}{n_1}+\dfrac{1}{n_2}\right)}}$$

Note. *In literature the criterion for the difference of the relative frequencies is often denoted as Z.*

THE CONFIDENCE INTERVAL FOR THE FRACTIONS DIFFERENCE OF NOT CONNECTED SAMPLES

Limits of the confidence interval for this case are calculated as follows:

$$\Delta p_{гранич} = \Delta p \pm t\overline{S}_{p_{1d}-p_{2d}}$$

Quantile of Student's t-distribution in case of a large sample with the significance level of 0.05 is considered to be equal to 1.96. When the sample is smaller, it is recommended to calculate it according to the Student's formula at different degrees of freedom.

If the confidence interval does not include zero, the null hypothesis is rejected, and the difference between relative frequencies can be considered to be significant at the given significant value.

3.4. ANALYSIS OF VARIANCE

Analysis of variance is the analysis of the variableness of the characteristic under the influence of some controlled variable factor. It is called ANOVA – "**ANALYSIS OF VARIANCE**". It allows identifying the cause-and-effect connection between variables.

The objective of analysis of variance is studying the importance of differences between means. It can seem strange but the procedure of comparing two means is called analysis of variance. In truth, it is connected with the fact that studying the statistical importance of difference between means of two (or several) groups, we actually compare (analyze) the sample variance. The fundamental concept of analysis of variance was proposed by R.A. Fisher in 1920. Maybe, the term "analysis of the sum of squares" would be more correct but owing to tradition it is

42

called "analysis of variance". Generally, the objective of analysis of variance is to mark out three particular variability of the total variability:
- Variability determined by the action of each of the studied independent variables;
- Variability determined by interaction between two studied independent variables;
- Random variability determined by all circumstances not taken into account;

Variability determined by the action of the studied variables and their interaction is associated with the random variability. The indicator of this correlation is Fisher's test.

TYPES OF ANALYSIS OF VARIANCE

Analysis of variance can be schematically subdivided into several types. This subdivision is carried out depending on the number of factors participating in the analysis, the number of variables influenced by the factors, the type of distribution, and the correlation between sampling values. Analysis of variance can be based on parametric and range tests. We will consider the one based on means comparison in samples, i.e. Fisher's exact test.

If *one factor*, which influence is being studied, is given, analysis of variance is referred to as *univariate*, and it is divided into two types:
- analysis of unconnected (different) samples;
- analysis of measured connected samples of the same group under different circumstances.

When simultaneous influence of two or more factors is being studied, we may speak of *multifactor* analysis that can be also subdivided according to its sample type. In this case the influence of each factor is calculated separately, as well as cooperative influence of the factors. We should point out that there is no a great difference between multifactor and univariate analysis. Multifactor analysis does not change a common logic of the analysis of variance, it just slightly complicates it, since apart from the estimating the influence of each factor separately on the dependent variable, we should estimate as well their combined influence. In this case the procedure of multifactor analysis using the computer is more economical, as it solves two tasks at one drive: it estimates the influence of each factor as well as their combined influence.

If several variables are subject to influence, we may speak of *multivariate* analysis. Multivariate analysis should be applied instead of univariate analysis only when dependent variables do not depend on each other but they correlate.

Restrictions of Fisher's ANOVA
- Analysis of variance should be applied only when it is specified that the distribution of the effective characteristic is normal.
- Each sample has to be independent of other samples.
- Each sample has to be randomly extracted from the population
- Variances of all samples have to be the same.

Note. *It is necessary to mention that F-test is stable to deviations from normality and homogeneity of variances.*

The analysis of variance for cases that go beyond these limitations will be considered later analyzing non-parametric tests.

Hypotheses formulation in analysis of variance

The null hypothesis H_0: means of the effective characteristic are the same in different conditions of the factor influence. The alternative hypothesis H_1: means of the effective characteristic are different in different conditions of the factor influence.

TEST CONSTRUCTION FOR THE ANALYSIS OF VARIANCE

Means difference of the measured values depending on the level of the acting factor (the dose of radiation, the type of temperament of the people being tested or the age of people being tested) can be expressed by the scatter of these means.

43

To estimate means difference, let us compare *intergroup means scatter* for m samples (or m levels of the operating factor) with the scatter of separate values inside each group (the number of the objects in each group is equal to n). Intergroup scatter can be calculated using this formula: $S^2_{intergroup} = nS^2_{\bar{x}}$ standard deviation of means $- S_{\bar{x}} = \sqrt{\dfrac{(\bar{x}_1 - \bar{X})^2 + (\bar{x}_2 - \bar{X})^2 + ...}{m-1}}$ Average value of sampling means for the group m is $\bar{X} = \dfrac{(\bar{x}_1 + \bar{x}_2 + ...)}{m}$

Intragroup scatter is $S^2_{intragroup} = \dfrac{s^2_1 + s^2_2 + s^2_3 + ...}{m}$

If the null hypothesis is true, the *intragroup* distribution as well as the *intergroup* represent the estimation of the same distribution σ^2, and should be approximately equal, and their ratio equals to 1. The more the intergroup scatter of means differs from the intragroup one, the less the probability of these groups being randomly sampled from the same population is. This is the reason why the test suggested by Fisher is calculated as follows:

$$F = \dfrac{\text{Variance of the population estimated on sampling means}}{\text{Variance of the population estimated on intragroup scatters}} \quad \text{or} \quad F = \dfrac{S^2_{intergroup}}{S^2_{intragroup}}$$

Test values that are bigger than 1 testify that there are no differences of means. In case of extracting samples from the normally distributed population, the test value will vary from one experiment to another. The critical value $F_{crit.}$ will depend on the significance value and the number of the degrees of freedom for intragroup and intergroup calculations.

If $F \geq F_{crit.}$, the null hypothesis at this significance value and these degrees of freedom $k_{inter} = m - 1$ and $k_{intra} = m (n - 1)$ is rejected, where m is the number of the groups (or factor levels), and n – the sample size. Taking into account that the degree of freedom has two values, and it is necessary to mark the significance value, the Fisher's tables of critical values are formed separately depending on the significance value (**Appendix 4**).

It is necessary to know that the quantitative gradation of the factor is not obligatory: the factor might have gradations not connected between each other by quantitative relations, and it can be represented even at the nominal scale. In general, we may speak not about the factor gradations but about different conditions of its action. The probability of quantitative gradation in this case is accidental. The researcher who wants to define the dependency of egg production capacity on the hen color can apply analysis of variance, choosing black, white and medley hen as the factor "color".

Note 1. Remember about the problem of multiple comparisons. Analysis of variance is just a common method of means comparing, and the Student's t-test is just a particular case. The advantages of the analysis of variance are the fact that it is far more effective (especially for little samples), and it also allows finding out the interaction of the factors.

It is possible that after the analysis and getting the significance value of p ≤ 0.05, pairwise (multiple) comparison of all groups (Post-hoc tests: Newman-Keuls method, Dunkan method etc) does not reveal statistically important difference in any pair. It is determined by the little potency of the pair-wise comparison tests. In such case Student's t-test for paired samples with Bonferroni adjustment can be used. For this it is necessary to establish the significance value 6 times smaller than 0.05 if the number of paired comparisons is equal to 6.

Post hoc (lat.) – after this.

Note 2. Algorithm of confidence interval construction for the mean value in each group and for the means difference of two groups after the pair-wise comparison is based on the formulae mentioned above.

CHAPTER 4

DEPENDENCE ANALYSIS

4.1. CORRELATION ANALYSIS

The final goal of any research or scientific analysis is to find a relationship between variables. Correlation or regression analyses are two ways to indentify the relationship between random variables.

The variables are dependant if their values systematically correlate with each other within the current observations. Height is connected with weight because usually tall individuals are heavier than the short ones. The number of mistakes in the test is connected with IQ, etc. The goal of statistics is to evaluate the relationship between the variables impartially.

The notion of function is used in mathematics to express the relationship between variables. It is reasonable to speak about functional dependence when a specific value of one variable correlates with a certain value of the other variable. In general this relationship is written as $y=f(x)$. For example, the relationship between circumference and the radius is linear: $L=2\pi R$. If $R = 1$ then $L = 2\pi$; if $R = 2$ then $L = 4\pi$, etc. In mathematics linear dependence is expressed as $y = kx + b$, where k is the angle of inclination to the straight axis x.

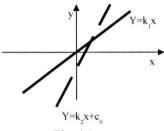

Fig. 4.1

However, in biomedical experiments usually one characteristic value corresponds to several *random* characteristic values. For example, people with the same height may have different weight, though there is the certain dependence between the means of these parameters.

The regularities connected with the random variables can be only statistical and, therefore, averaged in their nature. In relation to the specific object under observation, these regularities can be only approximate and probabilistic in their nature.

This kind of dependence between the random variables X and Y, where each their value does not correspond to the certain value, but to the specific group mean of the other value, is called **stochastic** (Greek 'stochasis' – random, probabilistic). In the XIX century a French paleontologist Léopold Nicolas Frédéric Cuvier formulated the law of correlation for animal parts and organs. This law allows us to reconstruct the body shape of an animal with the help of the found parts of the body. Later an English biologist Francis Galton introduced the term in statistics which meant not just *relation*, but *correlation*.

There are many examples of correlation. In medicine it can be the number of cold-related diseases per month in the medical district and the average monthly temperature; in sociology - the number of marriages per year, and the number of births the next year; in agriculture - the amount of precipitation and the yield on the fields; in pedagogic - the amount of reading material before an exam and the examination mark, etc.

Correlation analysis also helps to find out both the strength of the relationship between random variables, and its direction.

COVARIANCE COEFFICIENT

Before describing the correlation coefficient, let us consider the auxiliary quantity - the covariance coefficient.

The word "covariance" means "change together". The relationship between random variables means that the parameters X and Y are changing together to a great extent. This phenomenon is called covariance. As regards height and weight, probably a tall person has the bigger weight while a person with a height below the average has the lower weight.

To characterize the degree of covariance in mathematical statistics, covariance coefficient is introduced.

Covariance coefficient in the general population
It is denoted by the letter μ and calculated according to the formula:

$$\mu = \frac{\sum_{i=1}^{N}(x_i - a)(y_i - b)}{N} = \frac{(x_1 - a)(y_1 - b) + (x_2 - a)(y_2 - b) + ... + (x_N - a)(y_N - b)}{N}.$$

Here, a – mathematical expectation of the random variable X;
b – mathematical expectation of the random variable Y;
N – general population size.

The parameter μ is a mean product of deviation of two random variables from their means in the population. In other words, its essence is a mean covariance. Let us compare two cases to understand why μ reflects the presence or the absence of relationships between two variables.

1. Let us assume that there is a relationship between the random variables of *height* and *weight*, namely *the larger X is, the larger Y is*. So in the numerator of a fraction the terms of type (+)(+) and (-)(-) will prevail. Thus, if a person is taller than the general population $(x_i-a)>0$, the weight will be larger than the average weight $(y_i - b)>0$; and if he is shorter than average, his weight will be smaller than average, then the deviations of both height and weight will be negative. It is important that both of these terms are positive, and they are summarized. There will be such terms as (+)(-) if a person is tall and skinny, and there will be such terms as (-)(+) if a person is shorter than average and his/her weight is bigger than average. However, there will be considerably few terms of this type. That is why if they are negative, they decrease the positive sum that is formed by the prevailing objects of observation, but they cannot influence it considerably. As a result, if there is covariance, there will be a certain positive sum in the numerator of the fraction.

2. If there is no relationship or covariance, the terms of all four types in the numerator must occur with equal probability, as the concrete values x_i and y_i deviate from their original values a and b to the higher or the smaller sides independently from each other. Then the number of positive terms will be equal to the number of negative ones. In spite of the fact that all these terms will greatly vary in their values among different objects of observation, if there is a large number of the terms in the population, there will be zero in the numerator. That is why the result $\mu = 0$ shows that there is no relationship between random variables under observation.

There is one more good way to explain why the sum in the numerator and covariance coefficient μ will be 0, if there is no relationship.

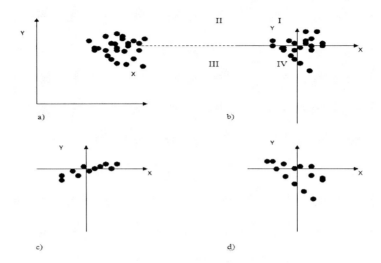

Fig. 4.2 Correlation cloud in different cases: a and b – with no relationship; c – with the straight relationship; d – with the inverse relationship

If the random variables X and Y are placed on two perpendicular axes lying within the plane, each object under observation with its x and y will produce a separate point (Fig.4.2 a).

The combination of these points is called correlation cloud. The center of such cloud is the point with the coordinates a and b. Points density is not the same in this cloud. The closer to the center it is, the higher the density is; the closer to periphery it is, the lower the density is, due to the fact that both variables have a normal distribution.

If origin of coordinates is in the center of the cloud (Fig.4.2 b), the points making up the cloud will spread out among four quadrants where in the points I and III there will be the positive terms in the formula for μ, and in the points II and IV they will be negative. That is why if both the square of all four quadrants of the cloud and points symmetrical density are equal, the numerator will be zero in the formula.

Covariance coefficient will not be equal to zero if correlation cloud is extracted or placed either in the I−III quadrants (then $\mu>0$, Fig.4.2 c) or in the II−IV quadrants (then $\mu <0$, and the negative sum will be in the numerator, Fig.4.2 d). The more extracted correlation cloud is, the larger the sum in the numerator is, and the stronger the relationship between random variables is. That is why the construction of the correlative cloud is a vivid and effective way to evaluate the presence of relationship between studied random variables.

Sample Covariance Coefficient

Sample covariance coefficient m_{xy} serves to evaluate the original value of the covariance coefficient. Proceeding from the population to the sample, let us make some certain changes in the variables' names and make a correction in the denominator, namely put 1 there. After this correction, μ evaluates the coefficient m_{xy} better.

$$m_{xy} = \frac{\sum_{1}^{n}(x_i - \bar{x})(y_i - \bar{y})}{n-1} = \frac{(x_1 - \bar{x})(y_1 - \bar{y}) + (x_2 - \bar{x})(y_2 - \bar{y}) + ... + (x_n - \bar{x})(y_n - \bar{y})}{n-1}.$$

Covariance coefficient is suitable when there is no the relationship between random variables. If it equals to zero, there is no the relationship. If there is the relationship, we can see its disadvantage which consists in the fact that covariance coefficient value depends on the measurement scale. If height is measured in meters, centimeters, etc., and weight is measured in kilograms, grams, milligrams, etc., the numerical values of μ (or m_{xy}) will be different. Consequently, it is impossible to say something about the strength of relationship relying on the absolute values of the numerals μ or m_{xy}.

CORRELATION COEFFICIENT

Correlation Coefficient in the Population
Correlation coefficient is denoted by the letter ρ, and it is obtained from the covariance with a help of normalizing standard deviation of both variables. The formula of transition from μ to ρ is as following:

$$\rho = \frac{\mu}{\sigma_x \sigma_y}.$$

Normalizing removes dimension, and the coefficient characterizing the *strength of relationship* becomes fractional and varies within the limits between 0 to ± 1. Correlation coefficient equals to zero when there is no relationships between random variables. It takes on the maximum value, namely 1, when the correlation relationship turns into the functional one, i.e. it becomes absolute or 100%. In this case the numeral 0.8 means that the strength of relationship between random variables is 80% from the absolute or functional one.

Thus, if one variable is increasing, the other is increasing as well, correlation is said to be *linear* and positive. If one variable is decreasing, the other is increasing too, and correlation is called *inverse,* and it is negative.

There are three ranges of absolute values for the correlation coefficient:
- 0-0.3 – low correlation (i.e. 30% of functional correlation);
- 0.3-0.7 – medium correlation;
- 0.7-1.0 – high correlation (over 70% of functional correlation).

If we put the formulas for μ, σ_x and σ_y into the formula, there will be the calculation formula for ρ:

$$\rho = \frac{\sum_{i=1}^{N}(x_i - a)(y_i - b)}{\sqrt{\sum_{i=1}^{N}(x_i - a)^2}\sqrt{\sum_{i=1}^{N}(y_i - b)^2}}.$$

Sample Correlation Coefficient
The true value of the correlation coefficient is estimated with the help of the sample correlation coefficient denoted as **r**.

Passing from the population to the sample, let us make up the necessary changes. We obtain the formula for the sample correlation coefficient which is called *Pearson correlation coefficient.*

$$r = \frac{m_{xy}}{S_x S_y}.$$

If we insert the formulas of the standard deviations into the formula, it looks as following:

$$r = \frac{\sum_{i=1}^{n}(x_i - \bar{x})(y_i - \bar{y})}{\sqrt{\sum_{i=1}^{n}(x_i - \bar{x})^2}\sqrt{\sum_{i=1}^{n}(y_i - \bar{y})^2}}.$$

48

TEST OF CORRELATION COEFFICIENT SIGNIFICANCE

It is common knowledge that the decrease of the sample size always decreases certainty and significance of the obtained figures. Small sample makes the significance of r more susceptible to randomness. The sample consisting of 3-5 people can both give the wrong numeral value of r and falsify the data about the relationship between the values. If 2 out of 3 individuals under observation have height taller than average, and weight lower than average, and the 3rd person is shorter than average, but heavier than average, thus, the correlation coefficient will be negative. We can conclude that there is an inverse relationship between height and weight, i.e. the higher the person is, and the lighter he/she is.

As the value of the coefficient r in the sample may differ from the value ρ in the population, it is necessary both to find out the value of r and check its significance. Having the values of the correlation coefficient and its error, it is possible to check the assumption that the coefficient equals to zero, i.e. to prove that there is no relationship between the parameters under observation. To test this hypothesis Quantile of Student's-t distribution with given significance value is used. In this case two hypotheses are made.

The main statistical hypothesis examined with the help of the correlation analysis is non-directional, and it asserts that the correlation equals to zero in the population H_0: $\rho_{xy}=0$. In case of its deviation the alternative hypothesis is accepted, namely H_1: $\rho_{xy}\neq0$.

Depending on the sign of the evaluated correlation coefficient, the correlation is either positive or negative.

On the basis of the acceptance or rejection of the hypotheses, the conclusions are made. If the results of the statistical test show that H_0 does not deviate on the level α, we conclude that the relationship between X and Y is not found. But if H_0 deviates on the level α, the conclusion is opposite, namely there is the positive (negative) relationship between X and Y. However, it is important to be very cautious about interpreting the correlation.

The main conceptual restriction of all the methods of regressive analysis consists in the fact that they allow us to identify only the numeric dependence, but not the causal relationship which is said to be their basis. For instance, Stanton A.Glanz [6] states that the research made by D.S. Drasar has found out that breast cancer occurs more often among women who have a high income level, and the number of cars and TV-sets. Thus, there is a relationship between the number of cars and the incidence of diseases. However, it does not mean that if a woman buys a car, she will get cancer. Probably, there is some hidden factor like diet which is rich in animal fats etc.

To check the hypothesis it is necessary to evaluate the correlation between the discovered value of the correlation coefficient and its standard error, i.e. where the criterion t is:

$$t = \frac{r}{S_{\bar{r}}}.$$

Having a big number of observations (n $\geq$ 100), the standard error of the correlation coefficient is identified with the help of the following formula:

$$S_{\bar{r}} = \frac{1-r^2}{\sqrt{n}}.$$

If the number of observation is less than 100, it is recommended using the other formula:

$$S_{\bar{r}} = \sqrt{\frac{1-r^2}{n-2}}.$$

After the change we obtain the formula for the small samples:

$$t = \frac{|r|}{\sqrt{1-r^2}}\sqrt{n-2}.$$

49

The null hypothesis is rejected for $t_{calc} \geq t_{crit}$ for $k = n - 2$, and the given significance level of α (or reliability level $P = 1 - α$). If $t_{calc} < t_{crit}$, the null hypothesis is accepted and the deviation of the sample correlation coefficient from zero is considered to be random.

For example, if $t_{calc} = 2.52$ and $n = 14$, the null hypothesis is rejected with the significance level of α = 0.05, as $t_{crit.} = 2.18$. However, when the significance level of α = 0.01, $t_{tab} = 3.05$. It means that we cannot guarantee that the hypothesis works in 99 cases out of 100, but it does in 95%.

CONFIDENCE INTERVAL FOR THE CORRELATION COEFFICIENT

If two variables are approximately normally distributed, the approximate confidence interval of 95% for ρ_{xy}:

$$\left(\frac{e^{2z_1} - 1}{e^{2z_1} + 1}; \frac{e^{2z_2} - 1}{e^{2z_2} + 1} \right),$$

where $z_1 = z - \dfrac{t}{\sqrt{(n-3)}}$, $z_2 = z + \dfrac{t}{\sqrt{(n-3)}}$, and $z = 0{,}5 \log_e \left[\dfrac{(1+r)}{(1-r)} \right]$.

Quantile t equals to 1.96, if the sample is large enough. If the sample size is less than 30, $t_{p,k}$ is placed in the table of Student on the line $k = n - 2$ (the number of degrees of freedom). Also it is possible to use a module *Probability Calculator* in the statistical software package Statistica.

If confidence interval contains zero, zero correlation coefficient cannot be present in the population with a high probability, i.e. the relationship between the characteristics exists in the population. In this case the correlation coefficient is statistically significant. If zero is in the confidence interval, zero correlation may occur in the population with a high probability, i.e. there is no relationship. In this case the correlation coefficient is statistically non-significant.

Note: *The calculation of the Pearson correlation coefficient between two variables is possible only when the relationship between them is linear (unidirectional). If the relationship, for example, has the U-shaped curves (multiple-valued), the correlation coefficient is improper for using it as a measure of relationship strength, thus, its value tends to become zero.*

ASSOCIATIONS

Association is the way of describing interdependence of the qualitative characteristics. The measure of association between them is a quantitative indicator of the relationship strength. Here crosstabulation tables are used.

Note: *Association does not imply a cause-effect relation. Perhaps, both values depend on some other value if they are associated with each other.*

4.2. REGRESSION ANALYSIS

The estimation of the correlation coefficient allows us to establish the strength of relations between the characteristics and its direction. However, it is impossible to find out how the varying characteristic changes on average when there is a change in the unit of measurement of the other characteristic connected with it. This problem is solved with the help of regression analysis.

Regression analysis allows us to estimate how one variable depends on another one, and what the scatter of the dependent variable values around the line determining the dependence. These estimations and corresponding confidence intervals predict the value of the dependent variable and find out the correctness of this prediction. Regression analysis describes the dependence between random variables with the help of regression (linear, quadric, etc).

Obviously, everyone uses regression analysis, when they try to define their weight Y with the help of the regression equation $Y = X - 100$, knowing their height X.

Regression is a function which allows measuring the average (expected) relationship between correlated characteristic value $\hat{y}_x$ and x.

Unlike the correlation coefficient, the parameters of regression are the denominate quantities.

Note: *A sign ^ denotes the estimated values.*

The regression equations that describe the dependence between random variables can be different. In this chapter we observe only linear regression that is expressed by the equation of linear dependence:

$$\hat{y}_x = bx + a_0,$$

where b is the angular coefficient, and a_0 is the absolute term.

The goal of regression analysis is to find the figures b and a_0. Then it is possible to insert various values of x and predict the corresponding to it the average values of $\hat{y}_x$. There are two regression equations. In the first x is an independent variable, and $\hat{y}_x$ is the dependent one, and it is called "Y on X". In the second, on the contrary, y is an independent variable, and $\hat{x}_y$ is the dependent one, and such equation is called "X on Y".

The main conditions for the linear regression model
- zero mathematical expectation of errors;
- bias of the covariance matrix of errors;
- absence of heteroscedasticity in the model.

Note: *Distribution of the random member of regression is homoscedastic, if variance remains permanent. Heteroscedasticity is the impermanence of variance.*

The violation of any of these conditions leads to falsification of the obtained results, i.e. there is a possibility not to identify the existing dependency or to make a wrong model. Though the method seems to be simple, it hides the whole complex of problems that are not obvious from the first sight.

Consider the relationship between two random variables, namely X (height) and Y (weight). As we deals with the sample, we will use the sample parameters.

In regression analysis the basis is the search for the "best fit" line, going through experimental points on the graph of the relation between the indicators X and Y.

To obtain this "best fit" line usually the least-squares method is used, and it allows us to choose the line, from which the sum of the distances to every point will be minimized. But as this method is complicated enough, we use the simpler way of explanation how to find this line.

Turn to the Fig.4.3a. Let us assume that there are two samples taken from the same correlation cloud. Assume that in the first sample all people out of 20 have the height x_1 which equals to 165 cm. In the second sample consisting of 20 people the height x_2 lies in the range of the bigger values, for example, everybody's height is 180 cm. All people can have different weight that is why the whole group of the values of weight, namely the points on the vertical axis, will correspond to each sample. The centers of these points are the average of $\bar{y}_1$ and $\bar{y}_2$ corresponding to the values of x_1 and x_2. A straight line goes through these points, and it is the graph of regression equation. In mathematics it is known that any line on the graph can be described by some equation (e.g. $y = x^2$, $y = \sin(x)$, $y = kx$, etc.). In this case the obtained straight line is described by the equation of linear dependency and is called "Y on X".

$$(\hat{y}_x - \bar{y}) = k_1(x - \bar{x}).$$

Proportionality coefficient is estimated by the formula:

$$k_1 = r\frac{S_y}{S_x}.$$

In the equation all parameters, except for x and $\hat{y}_x$, have the concrete figures. That is why if we insert all these figures, multiply them and gather all absolute terms together, we obtain the linear equation written as:

$$\hat{y}_x = b_1 x + a_{01}.$$

The slope coefficient b_1 of the regression line or the slope of the graph reflects the strength of relationship between the variables, as its values depend on the correlation coefficient r.

This equation makes it possible to find $\hat{y}_x$ by placing the known value x there.

On the graph of the other equation "X on Y" the algorithm remains the same (Fig.4.3b), namely two samples with a certain weight, for example, $y_1 = 65$ kg and $y_2 = 85$ kg, are chosen. Then the points of the distribution of height, corresponding to these two samples of weight, are built. After this the average values of $\bar{x}_1$ and $\bar{x}_2$ are defined, and then the line of the graph of the second equation "X on Y", going through these values, is drawn:

$$(\hat{x}_y - \bar{x}) = k_2(y - \bar{y})$$

Proportionality coefficient k_2 is estimated by the formula:

$$k_2 = r\frac{S_x}{S_y}.$$

After placing the known values and their rearrangement, we obtain an equation written as:

$$\hat{x}_y = b_2 y + a_{02}$$

This equation allows us to find $\hat{x}_y$ by placing the known value y there.

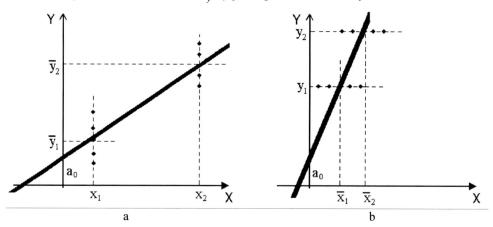

Fig.4.3 The principle of creating the regression equations: a: averaging Y; b: averaging X.

The regression equations show that the slope of the line for the created equations can be different (different coefficient next to variable). *So the asymmetry of regression analysis bothers us to use it straightly for description of the strength of relation.*

PREDICTED VALUES AND RESIDUALS

The line of regression expresses the best fit prediction of the dependent variable (Y) according to the independent variables (X). However, it is not typical of nature to be completely predictable, and usually there is a considerable scatter of the points under the adjusted straight line (as it is shown on the diagram of the scatter). Residual is the deviation of a separate point from the regression line (from predicted value). Residual distribution must correspond to normality, therefore it is important to analyze residuals and plot their graph to understand to what extent the regression equation describes the data under observation. As the residuals themselves can be of different signs and null each other. The sum of the squares of the residuals is used in the analysis, and it must be minimal.

The value $S_{x|y}$ is called the residual standard deviation (or the residual dispersion $S^2_{x|y}$). It is connected with the standard deviations S_y and S_x for dependant and independent variables.

$$S_{y|x} = \sqrt{\frac{n-1}{n-2}(S^2_y - b^2 S^2_x)}$$

There is the coefficient b in the regression equation with the variable x.

As the predicted values of the dependent variable are just the sample estimation of the data in the population, we need to estimate the errors in predictions, i.e. to construct the confidence intervals.

If it is necessary to predict not a particular value y, but its average value, the standard error is written as:

$$\bar{S}_{\hat{y}} = S_{y|x} \cdot \sqrt{\frac{1}{n} + \frac{(x-\bar{x})^2}{(n-1)\cdot S^2_x}} \cdot$$

If we want to predict the individual value y with the given value x, we need to remember that the standard error of y in this case is written as:

$$\bar{S}_{\hat{y}} = S_{y|x} \cdot \sqrt{1 + \frac{1}{n} + \frac{(x-\bar{x})^2}{(n-1)\cdot S^2_x}}$$

In contrast to the standard errors, $\bar{S}_{\hat{y}}$ with different x takes on different values. The further x from the sample average $\bar{x}$ is, the bigger it is.

The borders of the confidence interval for the true value of the regression equation in the point x can be estimated by the formula $t_{p,k} \cdot \bar{S}_{\hat{y}}$, and the critical value of Student's t Quantile can be found in the table for the given level of significance with the degrees of freedom $k = n - 2$.

According to these values we state that if there is a given value x, the true value y lies in the limits of the confidence interval with the given probability. The regression line for the predicted values of height relatively to the known values of weight goes in the middle (Fig.4.4), and the lines of the confidence intervals are drawn on both sides. With the specified probability, usually 95%, we can state that the true line is somewhere inside this range.

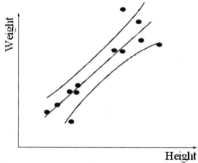

Fig. 4.4

Note that two points are outside the borders of the confidence interval. It is quite natural, as the interval is made for the regression line, but not for the values themselves. The confidence interval for these values will be much wider. If the separate values y are far out the borders of the confidence interval of the separate values, they are called outlying cases.

Note: *Outlying cases or extreme observations can cause a serious bias of estimators, "moving" the regression line in a certain direction and causing the bias of regression coefficients. Often the exclusion only of one extreme observation leads to the completely different result.*

COEFFICIENT OF DETERMINATION

Let us consider the other ways of estimating the quality of regression model. The quadric range of values of the dependent variable relative to the average can be divided into two sums:

$$\sum (y_i - \bar{y})^2 = \sum (y_i - \hat{y}_{xi})^2 + \sum (\hat{y}_{xi} - \bar{y})^2$$

They can be denoted as following: SS = RSS + ESS

$SS = \sum (y_i - \bar{y})^2$ - *Sum Of Squares* – the total sum of squares of the deviations of the observed values from the average value of the dependent variable;

$RSS = \sum (y_i - \hat{y}_{xi})^2$ - *Residual Sum Of Squares* - the sum of squares of the deviations of the observed values from the predicted values of the dependent variable; the "unexplained" sum of squares of residuals;

$ESS = \sum (\hat{y}_{xi} - \bar{y})^2$ the sum of squares of the deviations of the predicted values from the average value of the dependent variable; the regression sum of squares, also called the *Explained Sum Of Squares*

If the equation is divided both on the left and the right sides into SS, the relation ESS / SS is the estimation of the fraction of unexplained dispersion. The fraction of dispersion of the dependent variable, explained by a predictor that is included in the regression equation, is called the coefficient of determination. It is estimated as the difference between 1 (100%) and the fraction of unexplained dispersion.

$$R^2 = 1 - \frac{RSS}{SS}$$

The level of interdependence is estimated by using the coefficient of determination R^2. The closer to zero the second summand is, the closer R^2 to zero is, the better the regression model describes the data under observation. The root from the coefficient of determination is called the correlation coefficient. In the two-dimension case the correlation coefficient coincides with the root of the correlation coefficient r^2.

4.3. MULTIPLE CORRELATION AND REGRESSION

MULTIPLE CORRELATION DEPENDENCE

To change the correlation ratio in case of multiple correlation dependence (i.e. in case of study of two or more characteristics simultaneously), multiple and partial correlation coefficients are estimated.

Coefficient of multiple correlation is calculated when there is a linear relationship between the effective and several factorial characteristics (predictors), and also between each pair of the factorial predicators. For example, the multiple correlation coefficient for two factorial characteristics is estimated by the formula

$$R_{yx_1x_2} = \sqrt{\frac{r^2_{yx_1} + r^2_{yx_2} - 2r_{yx_1}r_{yx_2}r_{x_1x_2}}{1 - r^2_{x_1x_2}}},$$

where r_{yx_1}, r_{yx_2}, $r_{x_1x_2}$ are the paired correlation coefficients between the characteristics Y and X_1, Y and X_2, and also between X_1 and X_2.

Multiple correlation coefficients vary within the limits from 0 to 1, and it is definitely positive $(0 < R < 1)$. The closer R to one is, the stronger the linear association is.

Partial correlation coefficient r_{xy-z} is calculated when it is necessary to examine the assumption about the fact that the relationship between two variables X and Y does not depend on the influence of the third variable Z. Very often two variables correlate with each other only because they are both changed under the influence of the third variable. In other words, there is no relationship between the corresponding characteristics, but it occurs in the statistical interdependence under the influence of the common reason. When interpreting a partial correlation from the point of view of causation, one must be cautious because if Z correlates with both X and Y, and the partial correlation r_{xy-z} is close to zero, it does not mean that it is Z that the reason for the presence of X and Y.

For example, we can identify the negative correlation between the hair length and height in the population (short people have longer hair). This strange dependence disappears if the variable 'sex' is added into the equation of multiple regression. It happens because women are shorter and have longer hair than men in average. Thus, after the insertion of the predicator 'sex' in the equation, the relationship between the hair length and height disappears, as the hair length itself does not contribute to the prediction of height which is shared with the sex. I.e. after taking into account the variable 'sex', the partial correlation between the hair length and height equals to 0. In other words, if one value correlates with the other, it means that they both correlate with a third value or a combination of values.

MULTIPLE REGRESSION

When creating regression models, first of all, we question the type of the functional dependence characterizing the interdependence between the effective characteristics and several factorial characteristics. The choice of relationship must be based on the qualitative, theoretical and logical analyses of the studied phenomena. The forms of relationship can be different, but we want to consider the linear one.

In case of the linear relationship the experimental data may be approximated by the linear equation to the 16th degree of equation:

$$y = a_0 + b_1x_1 + b_2x_2 + \ldots + b_{16}x_{16},$$

where a_0, b_1, b_2.... b_{16} are the sought regression coefficients. The independent variables x_i in the equation are called predictors. In this case if $x_i = 0$, y_0 equals to the absolute term $(y_0=a_0)$. When data is processed electronically, it is quite simple to create an equation for 16 predictors.

Let us indicate the meaning of the coefficients in the linear equation of the multiple regression. The value b_i shows how much the effective characteristic y changes in average, if the variable x_i changes on the unit of measurement scale when the values of the other x_i are fixed.

Thus, the "pure" influence of each of the factors on the result is evaluated. For example, $b_1 = y_1 - y_0$, if $x_1 = 1$.

The coefficients of regression b_i do not correlate with each other directly, because they depend on the measurement units of x_i. To make these coefficients correlate with each other, all characteristics must be expressed in the standard scale. So, all the coefficients of regression are standardized by using their relation to their own standard deviations instead of the original variables. Thus, the last equation is written as following:

$$\frac{y}{\sigma_y} = a_0' + \beta_1 \cdot \frac{x_1}{\sigma_{x_1}} + \beta_2 \cdot \frac{x_2}{\sigma_{x_2}}$$

The equation of multiple regression plotted with the help of the standard characteristics is called standard multiple regression, and the corresponding coefficients of regression are called standardized or β – coefficients. The coefficients β_i shows on how many standard deviations (σ_Y) y changes if x_i increases on the one standard deviation σ_x, if the rest factors of the regression equation are permanent.

The factors can be compared not only on the basis of β – coefficients, but also on the basis of their participation in the explained variance. This method is widely used in practice. F-criterion helps to examine the accuracy and maintenance of conditions, which must agree with the initial data in the equation of multiple regression.

Irrespective of the concrete form of the used regression equation, the result of regression analysis is evaluated according the following criterion:

- Overall level of interdependence between the predicators and response;
- The importance of the participation of each predicator to its evaluation;
- Accuracy of prediction of the response values ad probable errors of their evaluation.

The overall level of interdependence is estimated from the coefficient of determination R^2. It is the part of variance of the dependent variable explained by the predictors which are included in the regression equation. The closer to 1 it is, the better the quality of the regression model is. The root from the coefficient of determination is called the coefficient of multiple determination. The closer R^2 to the coefficient of multiple correlation in its value is, the closer the regression line to the straight line is.

If there are many predicators, a step-by-step method is used in one of two variants:

- The straight one which consists in increase of the number of predictors from the minimal to maximum possible value, where there is a statistically significant correlation coefficient;
- The inverse one which consists in decrease of the numbers of predictors to minimal, where there is also a statistically significant correlation coefficient.

Note.

Note that non-correlatedness for the characteristics, which distribution is close to normal, leads to independence.

The number of the objects must be several times higher than the number of the characteristics to make the equation parameters statistically reliable.

The multiple regression tempts its user to include all the possible variables as predictors, hoping that some of them will be significant. It happens this way because the benefit is gained from randomness. We also face this problem when the number of observation is small. When examining the relationship, it is important to pay attention to the fact that predictors must not correlate with each other (no multicollinearity).

If the conditions of use of the linear regression model are violated, the general regression model is applied. In the statistical package it is denoted as GRM. The coefficients of such model will be different from the sought one for the linear regression model. It is caused by another method of estimation. To develop a general regressive model, the least-squares method is used, as it has the wider field of uses and allows us to develop good models even if there are no conditions mentioned above.

CHAPTER 5

THE APPLICATION OF STATISTICA SOFTWARE PACKAGE FOR QUALITATIVE AND QUANTITATIVE ANALYSES

5.1. COMPARISON OF THE GROUPS BY QUANTITATIVE ATTRIBUTE

5.1.1. PARAMETRIC AND NON-PARAMETRIC TESTS

While analyzing the data, the user of the Statistica package must have a good handle in the types of statistic scales, and while choosing the method, he/she must pay attention to the fact that the proper types of scales have been defined. Having classified the variables according to statistic scales, it is necessary to check the presence of proper distribution and to single out dependent and independent variables.

While setting variables for the analysis in the Statistica package, the variables are denoted either as *Dependent variable*, or *Independent variable*, or *Grouping variable.* For example, if in the experiment men and women are compared in relation to their weight, gender can be defined as an independent variable, while weight is a dependent variable. If the observed samples, namely the healthy and the unhealthy, are independent variables, the variables of weight and height will be dependent in these samples as their variations depend on the type of the group.

STRUCTURING, INSERTING AND CHECKING THE DATA

Before applying the statistical methods or drawing the plots, they should be structured, i.e. the gathered data should be presented in the form which is proper for its processing.

To structure the data, you should follow the next algorithm:
- To define the scale which the variables are related to;
- To set the codes of variables for the qualitative variables (for example, if the condition is satisfactory, set 1, if the condition is not satisfactory, set 0) and insert the data taking into account the codification table;
- To insert the original data into the package (while inserting the data, the Statistica can use the files of such programs as Excel and dBase);
- To check whether there are no mistakes and there is conciseness in the inserted data.

Now we can start the statistical processing of the inserted data. In the Statistica the variables (the columns) are denoted as Var1 and Var2 on default, and the rows are denoted as the Cases. Their analysis can be done only for the observation which has been grouped in a certain way. If descriptive analysis needs to be done for two samples, the values of the variables are inserted in the neighboring columns and renamed, and then the analysis can be started. If we need to make a test on differentiating some parameter (e.g. height) in two groups, in one of the columns named as the dependent variable in the first 10 lines (with $n = 10$) we insert the code of the group (e.g. Group 1), and in the following 10 lines of the same column we insert the code of the second group (e.g. Group 2). Then, we fill the second column named as the independent variable with the corresponding values.

STANDARDIZATION OF VARIABLES

If the scales are different, when one variable changes, for instance, in the diapason from 0 to 1000, and the second one changes in the diapason from 0 to 10, it is necessary to standardize the variables, because though the influence of the predicators on the dependent variable is factually equal, the coefficient for the second variable will be 100 times greater than for the first one. Estimating the mean of the variables and dividing the difference by the standard deviations of the variables, we obtain the non-dimensional variables, the coefficients of which will be equal, if their influence on the dependent variable is the same. In regressive analysis the Statistica package conducts standardization automatically.

DESCRIPTIVE STATISTICS

This type of analysis includes the creation of frequency table, the estimation of the statistical characteristics or the graphical representation. The frequency tables can be created for the variables which are related to the nominal scale and for the ordinal variables that have not so many categories. Median and both quartiles are more frequently estimated for the ordinal variables and those that do not relate to the interval scale, but obey the normal distribution. For variables related to the interval scale and obeying the normal distribution, the mean value and the standard deviation or the standard mistake are more frequently estimated. For variables, related to all statistical scales, a great variety of the plots can be drawn where such characteristics as frequency, mean values, etc., will be represented.

In Statistica p-level has different designations. The mark * denoting the degree of signification is applied in several cases.

$p > 0.05$ non-significant;

$p <= 0.05$ significant *;

$p <= 0.01$ very significant **;

$p <= 0.001$ maximally significant ***.

NON-PARAMETRIC TESTS

As it was underlined above, parametric methods have the greater sensitivity than the non-parametric ones. That is why the parametric method is chosen on default. The decision of applying the non-parametric method is justified if the following conditions are accomplished:

• There is a reason to consider that the distribution of the characteristic values in the general population does not correspond to the law of normality;

• There are some doubts on the normality of the characteristic distribution in the general population, but the sample is too small to judge about the distribution in the general population according to the sample distribution;

• The requirement of homogeneity of variance is not accomplished while comparing the mean values for the independent samples.

In practice, the advantage of non-parametric methods is especially noticeable when the data has extremely large or small values. However, if the volumes of the compared samples are very small (there are less than 10 observations), the results of applying the non-parametric methods can be treated only as preliminary. The structure of the original data and the interpretation of the results of using both non-parametric and parametric methods are the same.

While comparing the sample using the non-parametric tests, usually undirected statistical hypotheses are checked, when two-sided test is used. The applying of the one-sided alternative is possible, when one-sided test is used.

Non-parametric tests can be applied for the normal distribution of the values as well. But in this case they will have only 95% of power in comparison to the parametric tests.

RECOMMENDATIONS FOR CHOOSING THE STATISTICAL TESTS

Let us distinguish the tests according to the field of their use and represent them in the table 5-1. It shows that every parametric test has at least one alternative non-parametric test. Each of them goes into one of the following categories:

• tests of differentiating for independent samples;

• tests of differentiating for dependent samples;

• the estimation of the degree of dependence between the variables.

58

Table 5-1

The classification of the main methods
(Table of choosing tests)

Quantitative characteristic		Qualitative characteristic
Parametric test with normal distribution	Non-parametric test with another or unknown distribution	Tables of frequency or percents
Estimation of the mean values, standard deviations and standard mistakes	Estimation of median or mode, quartiles and interquartile intervals	
t-test	Wald-Wolfowitz; Mann-Withney-U-Test; Kolmogorov-Smirnov	χ^2-Yates corrected Chi-square (if the presence of expected frequency is >20) Fisher exact p (if the sum of expected frequency is <20 and (or) there is the expected frequency that is <5) z or (t)-test for parts (Yates corrected)
Paired Student t-test	Sign test; Wilcoxon test	McNemar test
Variance analysis (ANOVA)	Kruskal-Wallis test Median-tests	χ^2-Chi-Square
Variance analysis of the repeated values (ANOVA)	Friedman rank analysis of variance	Q-Cochran
Pearson linear correlation; Linear regression	Spearman rank correlation coefficient; Non-linear regression	Pearson Chi-Square; Fisher exact p; McNemar test; Phi-Square; Rank-bi-serial coefficient; Kendall τ-coefficient; Gamma coefficient; Logit-regression

Except for these simple statistical methods, there are also more complex methods of multidimensional analysis in which usually a big number of variables is used.

TEST OF THE CHARACTER OF DISTRIBUTION FOR NORMALITY

Except for two ways of testing the normality of distribution with the help of *Skewness and Kurtosis* observed in the chapter 2, tests of fit are used, and they have some limitations of the volume of the sample:

- For the χ^2 test, $n > 20$;
- For the Kolmogorov-Smirnov test and the Lilliefors test, $n > 50$;

- *Shapiro-Wilk's* W-test examines small samples where n < 50.[1]

Note 1: *While choosing the hypotheses, it is necessary to analyze carefully the data on the presence of outliers; otherwise the null hypothesis can be rejected by mistake.*

Note 2: *If it is necessary to describe the main tendency and variances in the sub-groups, the test for normality of distribution in these sub-groups should be done.*

5.1.2. THE USE OF THE STUDENT T-TEST FOR TWO INDEPENDENT SAMPLES

Example 5.1 [6]

S.L.Hale and his co-authors measured the diameter of the coronary vessel after taking the nifedipine and placebo. Does the data shown below give us the right to state that the nifedipine influences the diameter of coronary vessels?

1. Launch the Statistica program. As the volume of samples equals 11 units of observation, add one more case. To do this, choose *Cases-Add* on the toolbar.

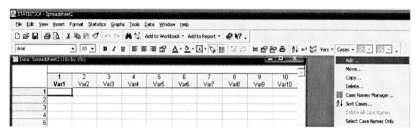

2. In the *Add Cases* window set '1' as the number of cases, and 'after 10 cases' as the place of insertion. Press **Ok**.

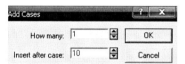

3. Denote the variables *Var1* and *Var2* as 'placebo' and 'nifedipine'. To do this, click twice on its headline *Var1*. The dialog window will be displayed. Insert 'placebo' instead of 'Var1' in the case *Name*. Then click the right navigation button and insert the name of the second column 'nifedipine'. Press **Ok**. Fill the columns.

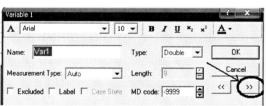

---

[1] In case, when the Lilliefors and Shapiro-Wilk's tests give different results, O.Y.Rebrova considers applying the Shapiro-Wilk's test as it is stricter than the first one.

	1 placebo	nifedipine
1	2,2	2,5
2	2,2	1,7
3	2,6	1,5
4	2	2,5
5	2,1	1,4
6	1,8	1,9
7	2,4	2,3
8	2,3	2
9	2,7	2,6
10	2,7	2,3
11	1,9	2,2

4. Test the normality of the sample with the help of **Shapiro-Wilk's W test.** The null hypothesis H_0 consists in the fact that the samples have been extracted from the general populations that have normal distribution of the examined features, and so, there is no difference between the normal distribution and the distribution of the examined samples. In the operation menu choose **Statistics – Basic Statistics/Tables.**

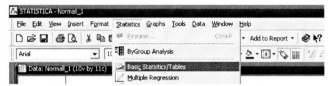

5. In the **Basic Statistics/Tables** window choose **Descriptive statistics**. Press Ok.

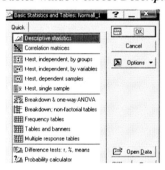

6. In the new **Descriptive statistics** window press the button **Variables**. Choose placebo and nifedipine. Press OK.

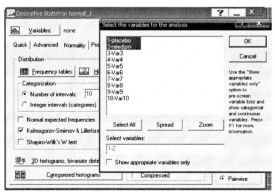

7. In the **Descriptive statistics** window choose the tag, set the option of the **Shapiro-Wilk's W test** and choose the tag **Quick.** Press the button **Histograms.**

61

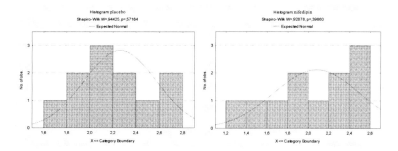

The **Shapiro-Wilk's W-test** has the significance larger than 0.05 for both cases. It allows us to accept the null hypothesis about the coincidence of distribution of the observed variables with the law of normal distribution for both samples. But there is skewness of distribution for nifedipine. Close the **Histograms** window.

Note: If at least one of two samples is extracted from the population with distribution that does not follow the law of normality, non-parametric test should be used for the following work with samples.

8. In the **Descriptive statistics** window choose the **Advanced** tag, set the options for obtaining the parameters of normal distribution, and choose the **Quick** tag. Press the button **Summary: Descriptive statistics**.

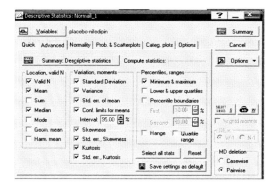

The analysis table will be displayed where the mean values and medians as well as the borders of 95% confidence interval for both features are shown. It is seen that the mean value and median coincide for placebo. The values of median and the mean values differ slightly from each other due to the skewness in the 'nifedipin' group. Close the table.

Variable	Valid N	Mean	Confidence -95,000%	Confidence +95,000%	Median	Minimum	Maximum	Variance	Std. Dev.	Standard Error	Skewness	Std.Err. Skewness	Kurtosis	Std.Err. Kurtosis
placebo	11	2,263636	2,054893	2,472379	2,200000	1,800000	2,700000	0,096545	0,310718	0,093685	0,146069	0,660687	-1,11927	1,279416
nifedipin	11	2,081818	1,803494	2,360142	2,200000	1,400000	2,600000	0,171636	0,414290	0,124913	-0,461190	0,660687	-1,11051	1,279416

Descriptive Statistics (Normall_1)

9. In the **Descriptive statistics** window choose the **Options** tag, set the option to display the mean value, standard mistake and maximum error **Mean/SE/1.96*SE,** and choose the **Quick** tag. Press the **Box&whisker Plot for all variables** button. The box-whisker plots will be displayed.

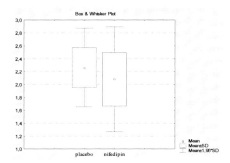

On the plot the mean values, the borders of the standard mistake and the borders of 95% confidence interval covering the real value and giving the data about the accuracy of the measurement will be shown. It is possible to obtain the data using the following options:

- *Median/Quartiles/Range*
- *Mean/SE/SD*
- *Mean/SD/1.96*SD*

Having assured that the distribution in both samples is normal, reorganize the data. Open the new worksheet in the Statistica. In the first column insert the diameter of the vessels, at first, for the placebo case, and then, for the nifedipine case. Name the column as *diameter*. Name the second column as *medicine*. Fill it with the names of variables. Use the functions of copying and autocompletion.

	1 diameter	2 medicine
1	2,2	placebo
2	2,2	placebo
3	2,6	placebo
4	2	placebo
5	2,1	placebo
6	1,8	placebo
7	2,4	placebo
8	2,3	placebo
9	2,7	placebo
10	2,7	placebo
11	1,9	placebo
12	2,5	nifedipine
13	1,7	nifedipine
14	1,5	nifedipine
15	2,5	nifedipine
16	1,4	nifedipine
17	1,9	nifedipine
18	2,3	nifedipine
19	2	nifedipine
20	2,6	nifedipine
21	2,3	nifedipine
22	2,2	nifedipine

1. In the operation menu choose the *Statistics – Basic Statistics/Tables – t-test, independent, by groups* section. Press Ok.

2. In the displayed *T-Test for Independent Samples by Groups* window press the *Variables* button, and choose *Dependent variables – diameter*, *Grouping variable – medicine*. Press *Ok*.

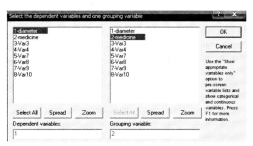

63

In the *T-Test for Independent Samples by Groups* window choose the *Options* tag and set the *Levene's test* option to test the equality of variances. Press the *Summary* button.

Variable	T-tests; Grouping: medicine (t_test) Group 1: placebo Group 2: nifedipine Mean placebo	Mean nifedipine	t-value	df	p	Valid N placebo	Valid N nifedipine	Std.Dev. placebo	Std.Dev. nifedipine	F-ratio Variances	p Variances
diameter	2,263636	2,081818	1,164445	20	0,257946	11	11	0,310718	0,414290	1,777778	0,378072

The displayed table shows that the null hypothesis about the absence of influence of nifedipine on the diameter of coronary vessels is accepted, as the level of significance is much higher than the critical one equaling 0.2579. Note that the *Levene's test* allows us to accept the null hypothesis about the equality of variances in the groups, as the level of significance is higher than the critical one equaling 0.2309 in this test. Close the table.

The construction of the confidence interval for the difference of real values is based on the formulas, reviewed in the theoretical part. Take the standard mistakes for both variables from the table of descriptive analysis (p.8). The value of the quantile of the t-Student can be found with the help of the *Probability calculator* module. To do this, in the operation menu choose *Statistics – Basic Statistics/Tables – Probability calculator*.

In the dialog window *Probability Distribution Calculator* choose the *t-Student* type of distribution, set the following options: *Inverse* – reverse function of the distribution; *Two-tailed* – two-sided test; the level of significance **1-Cumulative p** *(1-confidence probability)*. In the p-level window insert 0.05 (for 95% confidence interval). The number of degrees of variance *df*, in this case, equals 20 (11+11-2). Press the button *Compute*. The value of the quantile of t-Student will be displayed. It equals 2.085963 for these conditions.

5.1.3. THE USE OF T-TEST FOR TWO DEPENDENT SAMPLES

Assume that we need to know whether the chosen tactics cause the changes in basic cycle length of one and the same person before and after the arresting of congestive heart failure.

The algorithm of testing the null hypothesis is similar to the previous one. After the test for normality of distribution and descriptive analysis in the module *Basic Statistics/Tables* it is necessary to choose the *t-test, dependent samples* module.

5.1.4. COMPARISON OF TWO INDEPENDENT GROUPS WITH THE HELP OF MANN-WITHNEY U-TEST

Example 5.2 [6]
In the presence of retinal disease, the vascular permeability may increase. In 1986 G.Fishman and his co-authors measured the vascular permeability of retina among people who had this disease and those who were healthy. The obtained results are put in the table.

Table 5-2

Healthy	0.5	0.7	0.7	1.0	1.0	1.2	1.4	1.4	1.6	1.6	1.7	2.2
Unhealthy	1.2	1.4	1.6	1.7	1.7	1.8	2.2	2.3	2.4	6.4	19.0	23.6

It is necessary to check whether the differences of vascular permeability of retina are significant or not.

In this example it seems natural to use t-test. However, first of all, let us check the assumption about the normality of distribution of the features which is an imperative condition of using parametric t-test.

For doing this, we will use the *Shapiro-Wilk's W test* which is more proper for small samples. If the distribution turns to be far from the normal one, in the future we will use the corresponding non-parametric method.

Before statistical processing, let us formulate the statistical hypotheses.

The null hypothesis H_0 consists in the fact that the samples are extracted from the main populations having the normal distribution of observed features, and so, there is no difference between normal distribution and the distribution of examined samples.

The alternative hypothesis H_1 consists in the fact that the samples are extracted from the general populations in which the distribution of examined features differs from the normal one.

Analysis of the form of distribution of examined samples

1. Launch Statistica
2. To add observation, on the toolbar choose **Cases – Add…**
3. In the *Add Cases* window set 2 as the number of added cases, and 'after 10 case' as the place of insertion. Press Ok.
4. Denote the variables in the columns. In the case *Name* insert *(healthy)* instead of *Var1*. Then, click the right navigation button and insert (*unhealthy*) as the name of the second column. Press OK.

	1 healthy	2 unhealthy
1	0,5	1,2
2	0,7	1,4
3	0,7	1,6
4	1	1,7
5	1	1,7
6	1,2	1,8
7	1,4	2,2
8	1,4	2,3
9	1,6	2,4
10	1,6	6,4
11	1,7	19
12	2,2	23,6

5. Fill the columns. To test the character of distribution, in the *Statistics – Basic Statistics/Table* line of the operation menu choose the *Descriptive statistics.* Press Ok.
6. Press the *Variables* button. In the opened window highlight the variables named as healthy and unhealthy by mouse. Press Ok.
7. In the *Descriptive statistics* window choose the *Normality* tag. Choose *Shapiro-Wilk's W test.* Put off the other options, if they are set on default.
8. In the *Descriptive statistics* window press the *Histograms* button. Two histograms will be displayed. One of them is for the **unhealthy** group, and the other one is for the **healthy** group.

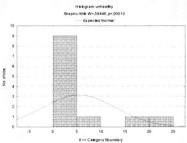

It is seen that in the unhealthy group the value of W-test equals 0.594, and the probability of the null hypothesis (regarding the fact that the distribution corresponds to the law of normality) equals 0.00010 or 0.01%. It is much lower that the critical level of significance 0.05 (5%). Thus, the null hypothesis is rejected. Besides, it is obvious that histogram is highly skewed, its peak is displaced to the left, and in the center there is an outlier.

As the distribution of the vascular permeability values of unhealthy people does not correspond to the law of normality, we should use the non-parametric **Mann-Withney W-test** to compare the values of factors of healthy and unhealthy people.

9.   In the bottom of the window choose the 'healthy' tag. The second diagram will be displayed:

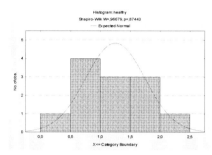

It shows that the value of W-test equals 0.967, and the probability of the fact that the observed distribution corresponds to the normal one, and it equals 0.874 that is much higher than the critical level of significance 0.5. Consequently, the alternative hypothesis is rejected. Besides, it is clear that the histogram is skewed enough, and its peak is placed closer to the center. Thus, the distribution of the values of vascular permeability of healthy people is close to normal (though the normal distribution itself is not the feature of health and medical norm!). Close the histogram. Let us proceed to the testing of hypotheses about the difference in retinal permeability. As it has been recognized that one of the samples does not obey the law of normal distribution, the non-parametric **Mann-Withney** U-test suits here for both independent groups that is the most sensitive in comparison to the other ones.

Mann-Withney rank-sum U-test is defined as the number of such pairs of x_i y_i that are not equal $(x_i > y_i)$, in other words, the zone of crossed values between two data sequences is small enough. The first sequence (the sample X) is called the one in which the values, according to the initial estimate, are greater, and the second sequence (the sequence Y) is the one in which the values are smaller. The smaller the field of crossed values is, the more possible it is that the differences are reliable. The empiric value of the U-test reflects how large the zone of coincidence between the sequences is. That is why the smaller the U_{emp} is, the more possible it is that the differences are reliable. U-test is the W-test extension for estimating which a single sequence of values of two samples is composed and ranged. Then, the ranged sequence is divided by two samples and the sum of ranks is counted in each sample. T_x is the greatest of the two rank sums corresponding to the sample with n_x objects. After this, the **Mann-Withney** U-test is estimated by formula:

$$U = n_1 \cdot n_2 + \frac{n_x(n_x + 1)}{2} - T_x,$$

Where n_1 is the volume of the first sample, n_2 is the volume of the second value.

Test limitations:
• The test is poorly applicable when there are many coinciding values in two samples.
• If the volumes of samples are great, the current test is approximated by the normal distribution.

Before statistical processing, let us formulate the statistical hypotheses.

The null hypothesis H_0: the retinal permeability of both healthy and unhealthy people is not different $(a_1 = a_2)$.

The alternative hypothesis H_1: the retinal permeability of both healthy and unhealthy people is different $(a_1 \neq a_2)$.

Work order

1.   To use **Mann-Withney** U-test it is necessary to set the data of two samples in one column and add the grouping variable, the values of which are the code marking the belonging of the data to the first or the second samples. To add the observations choose *Add.* in the toolbar. In the *Add* cases window set 12 as the number of added cases after the 12th case. Press *Ok*. The table 10×24 will be displayed. Then, highlight the data of healthy people by mouse and cut them with the help of contextual menu. Paste the cut fragment after the 12th case in the second column. Name the second column that contains the data of the dependent variable as *dependent.* Name the first column which will contain the codifying values of independent (grouping) variable as independent.

2.   Set the values of the grouping variable codes. To do this, insert **Unhealthy** for the values of unhealthy people in the first column (from the 1st to the 12th case), and **Healthy** – opposite to the values of healthy people (from the 13th to the 20th case). Use the function of autocompletion. Now the program can recognize the place of the data of healthy and unhealthy people. The fragment of obtained table looks as following:

	1 independet	2 dependet
1	unhealthy	1,2
2	unhealthy	1,4
3	unhealthy	1,6
4	unhealthy	1,7
5	unhealthy	1,7
6	unhealthy	1,8
7	unhealthy	2,2
8	unhealthy	2,3
9	unhealthy	2,4
10	unhealthy	6,4
11	unhealthy	19
12	unhealthy	23,6
13	healthy	0,5
14	healthy	0,7
15	healthy	0,7
16	healthy	1
17	healthy	1
18	healthy	1,2
19	healthy	1,4
20	healthy	1,4
21	healthy	1,6
22	healthy	1,6
23	healthy	1,7
24	healthy	2,2

3.   In the line of operation menu choose the *Statistics – Nonparametrics* section and highlight the *Comparing two independent samples (groups)*. Press *Ok*.

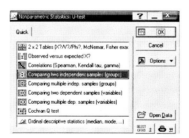

4.   In the displayed window press the *Variables* button. Then, set *Dependent variable list – dependent*, and **grouping variable-independent.** Press **Ok.**

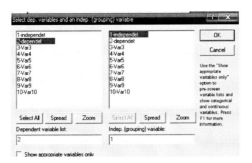

5. In the **Comparing Two Groups** window it is clear that the codes are automatically assigned to the groups of the same name. To carry out a test, press the **Mann-Whitney U test** button.

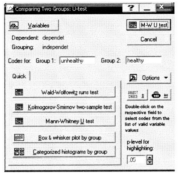

The table with the results of analysis will be displayed:

variable	Mann-Whitney U Test (U-test) By variable independet Marked tests are significant at p <,05000									
	Rank Sum **unhealthy**	Rank Sum healthy	U	Z	p-level	Z adjusted	p-level	Valid N unhealthy	Valid N healthy	2*1sided exact p
dependet	203,0000	97,00000	19,00000	3,059956	0,002214	3,070656	0,002136	12	12	0,001433

The Rank sums for each group and the p-level between these groups are estimated for the dependent variable. Using them, it is possible to answer the question whether the statistically significant values are observed or not. *p-level* (probability of the null hypothesis) equals 0.22%. Consequently, the alternative hypothesis stating that vascular permeability is different in the groups is correct.

To understand in which exact group the parameter is greater, it is necessary to compare the rank sum. It is bigger in the second 'unhealthy' group (203 vs. 97).

The essence of the parameters in the table: U is the value of **Mann-Whitney test;** Z is the corresponding value of the standard normal distribution test.

Thus, returning to the set objective, we should conclude that the difference of vascular permeability of retina (*U=19; p=0.002*) is statistically significant in the groups of both healthy and unhealthy people.

6.   To compare the differences visually, go back to the **Comparing Two Groups** window. To do this, close the window with the analysis table. Press the **Box&whisker plot by group** button. In the window where you can choose the variables, highlight two variables with the help of the mouse. Press **Ok**. The **Boxplot by Group** diagram will be displayed. On this diagram the difference between median, interquartile range and the diapason of changes of compared groups (Min–Max) is clear.

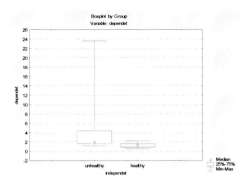

5.1.5. THE COMPARISON OF SEVERAL ORDERED GROUPS BY BINARY ATTRIBUTES WITH THE HELP OF THE MANN–WHITNEY TEST.

If there is a need to compare relative frequencies in several ordered groups, the **Mann–Whitney** test is used backwards: the binary attribute is taken as a *grouping* variable, while the *grouping* feature is analyzed as a dependent one. For instance, relative frequencies in the groups with the brain injury risk factor should be compared, if the influence of this factor on disseminated sclerosis is examined. Consider three groups of patients with I, II, III stages of the disease. Denote **Group category** as a dependent variable and the dichotomous variable **Trauma** (*yes*-1, *no*-0) as an independent one.

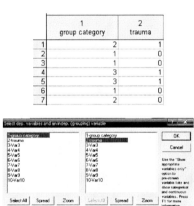

	1 group category	2 trauma
1	2	1
2	1	0
3	1	0
4	3	1
5	3	1
6	1	0
7	2	0

Mann-Whitney U Test (Gruppen)
By variable trauma
Marked tests are significant at p <,05000

variable	Rank Sum Group 1	Rank Sum Group 2	U	Z	p-level	Z adjusted	p-level	Valid N Group 1	Valid N Group 2	2*1sided exact p
group category	17,50000	10,50000	0,500000	1,944544	0,051831	2,057912	0,039599	3	4	0,057143

5.1.6. THE WALD-WOLFOWITZ TEST

The application conditions of this method are the same as for *the Mann–Whitney U test* or for the **Kolmogorov-Smirnov** test. The values of both groups range in a sequence, according to ranks. Then, the changes of the grouping feature which helps to determine the number of continuous sequences (the number of changes plus 1) are calculated. If there similar values (rank bonds) appear, the minimum and maximum values of possible continuous sequences are displayed. Based on the number of continuous frequencies, the probability error *p* can be determined. This test is not applicable to the variables with the small number of categories, as in this case the amount of rank bonds increases significantly.

5.1.7. THE COMPARISON OF CONTINUOUS QUANTITIES OF TWO RELATED SAMPLES WITH THE HELP OF THE W-WILCOXON TEST

The **W-Wilcoxon** test is a traditional nonparametric test to compare two dependent samples. This is the analogue of the parametric paired Student test. It is based on the arrangement of rank sequences of the absolute pair differences and is not limited by normal distribution. However, the variables should be measured at least on an ordinal scale. The value of the feature change is calculated for every patient. All changes are arranged by values (the sign is not taken into account). Then, the sign of the change (either plus or minus) is added to ranks. The values are summarized to obtain the **W** test. It allows identifying not only the direction of change, but also its degree. More specifically, it can determine whether the indicators' shift in one direction is more intensive than in the other. If the shifts do not differ much from each other, there is no sense in ranging a great amount of the same ranks. Similar results can be obtained with the help of the sign test.

Example 5.3.[6]. Is tensaprost effective as a diuretic?

The antihypertensive drug tensaprost measuring the activity of the prostaglandin system of vessel wall and having many side effects including diuretic activity is widely used in the therapy department. Therefore, some doctors assign tensaprost as a diuretic to the patients with the nephritic edema stating that it is rather effective. The resident medical practitioner has checked whether tensaprost is effective as a diuretic or not.

Six patients suffering from the hypertensive disease with nephritic edema were taking tensaprost.

Table 5-3

Patient's №	Daily diuresis		Diuresis measurements	Change rank	Sign rank
	Before treatment	After treatment			
1	1490	1600	110	5	5
2	1300	1850	550	6	6
3	1400	1300	-100	4	-4
4	1410	1480	70	3	3
5	1350	1410	60	2	2
6	1000	1050	50	1	1
Average	1325	1448	123		W=13

The table has shown that five patients have diuresis increased. But does it mean that the medicine is a diuretic?

Before starting statistical analysis let us formulate statistical hypotheses.

The null hypothesis H_0: diuresis has not been changed within the process of treatment.

The alternative hypothesis: H_1: diuresis has been changed within the process of treatment.

First of all, let us check the assumption about the normalcy of separate diuresis differences distribution which is an obligatory condition of the parametric paired Student's t-test application. Use the ***Shapiro-Wilk*** test to check up for normal distribution. If the distribution is far from being normal, the corresponding nonparametric method will be used in the future.

Work order

1. Launch the ***Statistica*** program.

2. Denote the columns. Put the first variable as ***before treatment***, the second as ***after treatment*** and the third as ***difference***. Press ***OK***. Enter the data to make a table:

1 before treatment	2 after treatment	3 difference
1490	1600	110
1300	1850	550
1400	1300	-100
1410	1480	70
1350	1410	60
1000	1050	50

3. Check up the distribution of differences which is indicative of the normalcy of distributions in samples. Choose *Statictics*, the *Basic Statistics/Table* section in the option menu. Click *Descriptive statistics* in a new window and press *OK*.

4. Click the *Normality* tab in the *Descriptive statistics* window and choose *Shapiro-Wilk's W test*.

5. Click *Variables*. Choose the *difference* variable in the opened window and press *OK*. Press *Histograms* to display the following histogram:

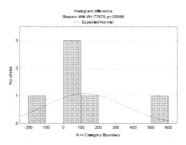

The histogram indicates that the value of W-test equals 0.77679 and the level of significance constitutes 0.03598 (3.6%). It is below the critical level making 0.05 (5%); therefore, the null hypothesis is rejected, and the alternative hypothesis saying that the distribution is far from being normal is accepted. Besides, it is obvious that the histogram has two outliers.

Thus, the distribution of the diuresis differences does not correspond to the normal distribution law. Hence, nonparametric test should be used to compare the diuresis. Moreover, the choice in favor of nonparametric test is determined by the small sample volume ($n=6$). Close the window with the histogram.

6. Choose *Statistics – Nonparametrics* and click *Comparing two dependent samples (variables)* to analyze the data. Press *Ok*.

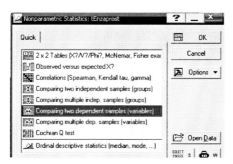

7. Press the *Variables* button in the opened window *Comparing two variables*. Then select *First variable list – Before treatment* in the left side of the window and *Second variable list – After treatment* in the right side of the window. Click *Ok*.

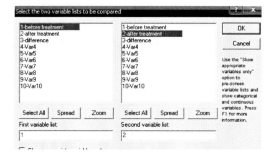

8. Click the ***Wilcoxon matched pairs test*** button.

	Wilcoxon Matched Pairs Test (tEnzaprost) Marked tests are significant at p <,05000			
Pair of Variables	Valid N	T	Z	p-level
before treatment & after treatment	6	4,000000	1,362770	0,172956

The table shows that ***p-level***, which is the probability for the absence of the diuresis changes or the probability of the null hypothesis, equals 0.173 (17.3%). This is much higher than the critical significance level 0.05.

Hence, the null hypothesis should be accepted. It can be concluded that tensaprost does not significantly influence (T=4.00; *p*=0.173) the daily diuresis, despite the fact that after taking the medicine the average diuresis increased by 123 ml (by 9.2%).

Close the table and return to the ***Comparing two variables*** window to evaluate the data analysis visually. Click the ***Box&whisker plot by group*** button, choose the variables ***before treatment*** and ***after treatment***, click ***OK*** and set the ***Median / Quart /Range*** option in the appeared window ***Box-Whisker Type,*** because the distribution is abnormal. Press ***OK***.

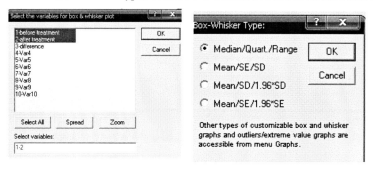

The ***Box&Whisker Plot*** window will be displayed.

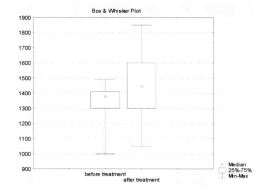

72

5.1.8. ONE-WAY ANOVA TEST

Example 5.4.

There is a necessity to identify the statistical significance of the *A* factor influence (with different levels of the factor) on the level of cystin in the blood plasma (mg/l). The measurement results at five levels of the factor *A* are listed in table 5-4

Table 5-4

*A*1	*A*2	*A*3	*A*4	*A*5
3.2	2.6	2.9	3.7	3
3.1	3.1	2.6	3.4	3.4
3.1	2.7	3	3.2	3.2
2.8	2.9	3.1	3.3	3.5
3.3	2.7	3	3.5	2.9
3	2.8	2.8	3.3	3.1

Let us state statistical hypotheses.

The null hypothesis H_0: there is no difference in the mean value of cystin between the groups (there is no influence of the factor *A*).

The alternative hypothesis H_1: the differences in the mean cystin level in the groups are statistically significant. It will be indicative of the influence of the *A* factor on the cystin level.

Work order

1. Launch the program **Statistica**.

2. Add **Cases** and enter 30 values of cystin in the first column out of five columns with different values of the factor *A*. Denote the first variable as cystin (it will depend on the factor *A*) and the second variable as **level *A***. Enter the numbers of the *A* factor levels. **A** part of the window is the following:

	1 cystin	2 level A
1	3,2	A1
2	3,1	A1
3	3,1	A1
4	2,8	A1
5	3,3	A1
6	3	A1
7	2,6	A2
8	3,1	A2
9	2,7	A2
10	2,9	A2
11	2,7	A2
12	2,8	A2
13	2,9	A3
14	2,6	A3
15	3	A3
16	3,1	A3
17	3	A3
18	2,8	A3

3. There are two ways to carry out the one-way ANOVA test. Let us consider one of them. Choose **Statistics – Basic Statistics/Tables – Breakdown & one-way ANOVA** in the option menu. Click **OK**.

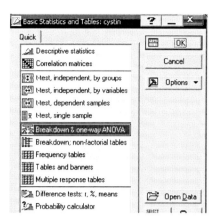

4. Click the *Individual Tables* tab in the appeared *Statistics by Groups (Breakdown)* window, press the *Variables* button to select the variables and enter *Dependent variable* as cystin and *Grouping variables* as *level A*. Press *OK*.

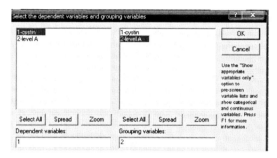

5. The normal distribution of the feature and the equality (homogeneity) of variance in groups are the conditions to carry out the parametric analysis of variance. It is examined by *Levene's test*. Click the *Lists of Tables* tab in the *Statistics by Groups (Breakdown)* window and set the options: *Levene test, Analysis of variance, Std. err. of mean* (standard error of the mean), *Conf. limits for mean (*confidence interval for the mean*)*, etc. Press the *Individual Tables*   tab and *OK*.

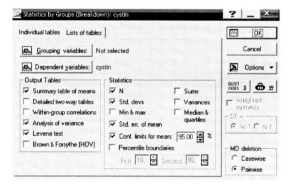

6. The analysis table will be displayed. Choose the tab *ANOVA&tests*. Click the button *Levene tests* to examine the equality of variances.

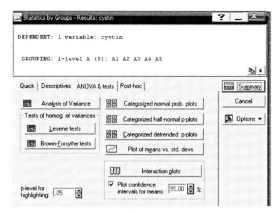

The analysis table of Levene's tests will be shown.

	Levene Test of Homogeneity of Variances (cystin) Marked effects are significant at p < ,05000							
Variable	SS Effect	df Effect	MS Effect	SS Error	df Error	MS Error	F	p
cystin	0,013926	4	0,003481	0,285370	25	0,011415	0,304997	0,871854

As the significance level of Levene's test is higher than critical 0.87, it allows accepting the null hypothesis which suggests the homogeneity of variances and the possibility to carry out parametric analysis of variance. Close the table.

7. Click the **Analysis of Variance** button in the **Statistics by Groups-Results** window to observe the table with the data of the variance analysis.

	Analysis of Variance (cystin) Marked effects are significant at p < ,05000							
Variable	SS Effect	df Effect	MS Effect	SS Error	df Error	MS Error	F	p
cystin	1,342000	4	0,335500	0,896667	25	0,035867	9,354089	0,000092

The level of significance 0.000092 is below critical that rejects the null hypothesis about the homogeneity of the means and accepts the alternative hypothesis. The carried out analysis has shown the difference between the cystin values at different *A* factor levels. To put it in other words, the influence of the A factor on the cystin level has been identified. Close the window.

8. Turn back to the **Statistics by Groups-Results** window, click the **Quick** tab and the **Interaction plots** button to observe the graphical representation of sampling data with key parameters. The mean values at every level of the acting *A* factor are denoted as dots and connected by a jogged line between each other. It is clear that the mean values of cystin differ from each other. Close the plot.

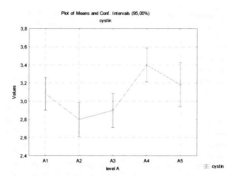

Press the *Descriptives* tab in the *Statistics by Groups-Results* window. Set the necessary options to obtain the descriptive group statistics. Click *OK*.

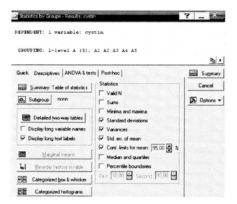

The displayed analysis table will indicate the mean values of cystin for every discrete group as well as for five groups collectively. The 95% confidence limits are identified.

5.1.9. POST HOC GROUP COMPARISONS

It should be kept in mind that the analysis of variance does not answer the question the difference between which groups is statistically significant. For this reason, pairs of groups should be compared using the Student test with the Bonferroni correction, which has been reported about in the theoretical part. It is made automatically in the *Statistica* program while carrying out *post hoc* comparisons in the *Post-hoc* sub module. *Post hoc* is derived from Latin and means *"after this"*. The term *a posteriori probability* means *after the event or experiment,* as the pair-wise comparison is carried out after the basic analysis of variance identifying the differences in general. Having used any of these tests, the level of significance makes it possible to say whether there are any differences between groups or not.

Work order

1. Return to the *Statistics by Groups-Results* window and click the *Post-hoc* tab. Carry out the pair-wise comparison between the groups. Press the *LSD test or planned comparison* button.

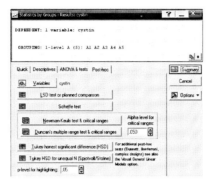

2. The analysis table which shows that there are statistically significant differences between the mean values of cystin for the *A1* and *A2*, *A4* levels, between *A2* and *A4*, *A5* and between *A5* and *A3*. All significance levels which are below 0.05 are marked by red. Close the window.

level A	LSD Test; Variable: cystin (cystin) Marked differences are significant at p < ,05000				
	{1} M=3,0833	{2} M=2,8000	{3} M=2,9000	{4} M=3,4000	{5} M=3,1833
A1 {1}		0,015735	0,106063	0,007739	0,369157
A2 {2}	0,015735		0,369157	0,000011	0,001740
A3 {3}	0,106063	0,369157		0,000113	0,015735
A4 {4}	0,007739	0,000011	0,000113		0,058627
A5 {5}	0,369157	0,001740	0,015735	0,058627	

Unfortunetely, this module has not the option to determine the confidence intervals for the difference of the means, but the *ANOVA/MANOVA* module has.

Consider another way to carry out one-way ANOVA test in *Statistica*.

Work order

1. Choose *Statistics –ANOVA* in the options menu. The type of analysis is *One-Way ANOVA*, the method of specification is *Quick specs dialog*, click OK.

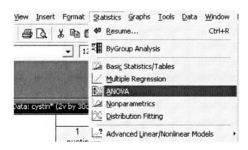

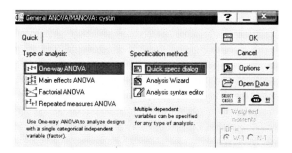

2.   Click *Variables* in the *ANOVA/MANOVA One-Way ANOVA* window. Choose *Dependent variable list – cystin, Categorical predictor (factor) – level A* and click *OK*.

3. Press *OK* in the *ANOVA/MANOVA One-Way ANOVA* window.

4.   The level of significance equals 0.05 by default in the *ANOVA Results* window (at the bottom of the window). Press *More results* there.

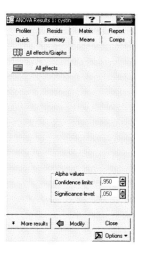

5.   The extended *ANOVA Results* window will be displayed. Click the *Assumptions* tab and *Histograms* in the group *Distribution of variables within groups*. Set the *All Groups* option in the appeared window where the variables can be chosen and click *OK*.

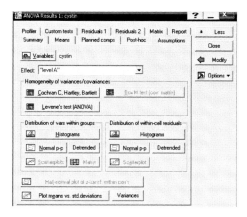

The normal distribution of the cystin variable can be assumed based on the plot. Close the plot and click *Histograms* in the group *Distribution of within-cell residuals*. According to the plot, the distribution coincides with the red line of normal distribution. It makes it possible to identify the parametric value of variance. Close the plot.

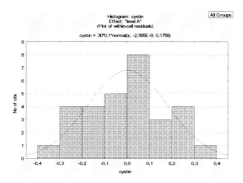

6.   Click the **Assumptions** tab in the extended **ANOVA Results** window. Choose **Levene's test (ANOVA)** and be sure in the homogeneity of variances ($p=0.871854>0.05$). It also serves as a ground to carry out the parametric analysis of variance. Close the windows of the analysis.

Levene's Test for Homogeneity of Variances (cystin) Effect: "level A" Degrees of freedom for all F's: 4, 25			
	MS Effect	MS Error	F	p
cystin	0,003481	0,011415	0,304997	0,871854

7.   Click the **Less** button in the extended **ANOVA Results** window. Press the button **All effects/Graphs** in the initial window **ANOVA Results** to display the table with the analysis results.

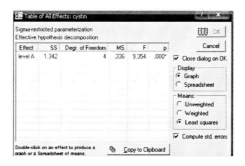

The table shows that the value of Fisher's test equals 9.354 and the level of significance makes 0.000*. Hence, the null hypothesis is rejected and the alternative one which states that the *A* factor influences the level of cystin is accepted. Close the window.

8.   In order to compare the difference visually, click the line containing the analysis results twice in the opened window. The graphical representation of sampling data with basic parameters will appear.

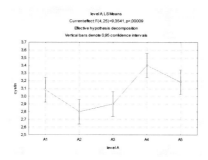

level A LS Means
Current effect F(4,25)=9,3541, p=,00009
Effective hypothesis decomposition
Vertical bars denote 0,95 confidence intervals

9. Close the tables with the results and click the **More results** button in the **ANOVA Results** window to carry out pair-wise comparison.

10. Press the **Post-hoc** tab in the extended **ANOVA Results** window. Set the **Significant differences** option in the **Display** group of options. Click **Bonferroni**.

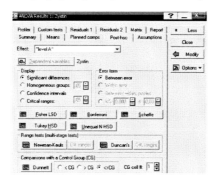

The analysis table will be shown.

Cell No.	level A	Bonferroni test; variable cystin (cystin) Probabilities for Post Hoc Tests Error: Between MS = ,03587, df = 25,000				
		{1} 3,0833	{2} 2,8000	{3} 2,9000	{4} 3,4000	{5} 3,1833
1	A1		0,157353	1,000000	0,077386	1,000000
2	A2	0,157353		1,000000	0,000106	0,017398
3	A3	1,000000	1,000000		0,001128	0,157353
4	A4	0,077386	0,000106	0,001128		0,586267
5	A5	1,000000	0,017398	0,157353	0,586267	

The mean values of cystin are listed in the line right under the title in every out of five columns of the initial table (3.0833; 2.8000; 2.9000; 3.4000; 3.1833). The levels of significance are indicated in the intersections of lines and columns. Those which are marked by red indicate statistically significant difference, as they are less than 0.05. The interjections of the columns *A2* with *A4* and *A5* as well as the columns *A3* and *A4* represent these data. Discordance with **LSD test** is explained by the fact that the **Bonferroni test** is more precise. Close the window.

11. Set the **Confidence intervals** option in the **Display** group of options of the **Post-hoc** tab in the extended **ANOVA Results** window. Click **Bonferroni**, after that the table containing the confidence intervals of the mean values difference for pair-wise comparison will be displayed. For instance, the difference between the groups *A2* and *A4* has made (2.8 - 3.4)=-0.6. The confidence interval for the difference ranges from -0.936 to -0.263. As far as the confidence interval does not take the null into account, the alternative hypothesis about the existence of differences with the significance level 0.05 should be accepted.

Cell No.	Bonferroni test; variable cystin (cystin) Simultaneous confidence intervals Error: Between MS = ,03587, df = 25,000					
	versus Cell No.	Mean Differ.	Standard Error	p	-95,00% LSD CL	+95,00% LSD CL
1	2	0,283333	0,109341	0,157353	-0,053241	0,619908
	3	0,183333	0,109341	1,000000	-0,153241	0,519908
	4	-0,316667	0,109341	0,077386	-0,653241	0,019908
	5	-0,100000	0,109341	1,000000	-0,436575	0,236575
2	3	-0,100000	0,109341	1,000000	-0,436575	0,236575
	4	-0,600000	0,109341	0,000106	-0,936575	-0,263425
	5	-0,383333	0,109341	0,017398	-0,719908	-0,046759
3	4	-0,500000	0,109341	0,001128	-0,836575	-0,163425
	5	-0,283333	0,109341	0,157353	-0,619908	0,053241
4	5	0,216667	0,109341	0,586267	-0,119908	0,553241

Note. Keep in mind the fact that clinical and statistic differences may diverge.

12.   Click the **Summary** tab and the **Coefficients** button in the extended window *ANOVA Results* to observe the table where weights of levels are specified. The universal mean 3.07 is indicated in the first line and the first column. In order to obtain the mean value of every example level, the corresponding coefficient should be added. For , the mean value for the level *A4* will be 3.07 + 0.32 = 3.4.

Effect	Parameter Estimates (cystin) Sigma-restricted parameterization											
	Level of Effect	Column	cystin Param.	cystin Std.Err	cystin t	cystin p	-95,00% Cnf.Lmt	+95,00% Cnf.Lmt	cystin Beta (?)	cystin St.Err.?	-95,00% Cnf.Lmt	+95,00% Cnf.Lmt
Intercept		1	3,073333	0,034577	88,88424	0,000000	3,002121	3,144546				
level A	A1	2	0,010000	0,069154	0,14461	0,886182	-0,132425	0,152425	0,023152	0,160107	-0,306694	0,352899
level A	A2	3	-0,273333	0,069154	-3,95255	0,000560	-0,415758	-0,130909	-0,632832	0,160107	-0,962579	-0,303085
level A	A3	4	-0,173333	0,069154	-2,50650	0,019063	-0,315758	-0,030909	-0,401308	0,160107	-0,731055	-0,071561
level A	A4	5	0,326667	0,069154	4,72378	0,000076	0,184242	0,469091	0,756312	0,160107	0,426565	1,086058

5.1.10. TWO-WAY ANOVA TEST

Consider how the problem about the influence of the medicine dose and the age of the examined person on the resulting factor can be solved.

Example 5.5. The influence of age and medicine dose on the medicine plasma exposure

Depending on age and medicine dose, 8 people were examined for some substance in the blood plasma (the variable *Analysis*). The significance of age and dose on the *Analysis* is to be evaluated. The initial data are listed in Table 5-5.

Table 5-5

№	age	dose		
		level 1	level 2	level 3
1	till 30 years	26	41	36
2	till 30 years	14	82	87
3	till 30 years	41	26	39
4	till 30 years	16	86	99
5	after 30 years	51	39	42
6	after 30 years	35	114	133
7	after 30 years	96	104	92
8	after 30 years	36	92	124

Suggest statistical hypotheses.

The null hypothesis H_0: the medicine dose and age do not influence the examined parameter.

The alternative hypothesis H_1: the medicine dose and age influence the examined parameter *Analysis*.

The fact that in this case the variables **Dose** and **Age** are referred to independent variables and the examined parameter is a dependent one should be paid attention to.

Work order

1. Launch the **Statistica** program.

2. Add the lines – **Cases**. Enter the variables. Denote the first variable as **Age** which is subdivided into two ranges. The second variable **Dose** is divided into 6 ranges. Denote the dependent variable as **Analysis**. The analysis window will look like this:

	1 age	2 dose	3 analysis
1	till 30 years	level 1	26
2	till 30 years	level 1	14
3	till 30 years	level 1	41
4	till 30 years	level 1	16
5	till 30 years	level 2	41
6	till 30 years	level 2	62
7	till 30 years	level 2	26
8	till 30 years	level 2	86
9	till 30 years	level 3	36
10	till 30 years	level 3	87
11	till 30 years	level 3	39
12	till 30 years	level 3	99
13	after 30 year	level 1	51
14	after 30 year	level 1	35
15	after 30 year	level 1	96
16	after 30 year	level 1	36
17	after 30 year	level 2	39
18	after 30 year	level 2	114
19	after 30 year	level 2	104
20	after 30 year	level 2	92
21	after 30 year	level 3	42
22	after 30 year	level 3	133
23	after 30 year	level 3	92
24	after 30 year	level 3	124

3. Choose **Statistics – ANOVA** in the option menu. Select **Factorial ANOVA – Quick specs dialog** in the appeared window to carry out two-way ANOVA test with repetitions. Press **OK**.

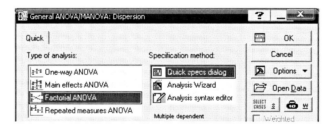

4. Click **Variables** in the **ANOVA/MANOVA Factorial ANOVA** window. Denote **Dependent variable list** as **analysis** and **Categorical predictors (factors)** as **age** and **dose**. Press **OK**.

5. Click OK in the **ANOVA/MANOVA Factorial ANOVA** window.

6. Press **More results** in the new window **ANOVA Results**. The level of significance equals 0.05 by default.

The extended **ANOVA Results** window will appear. Click the **Assumptions** tab in the **Effect** field, choose **age** and **dose** and press the **Levene's test (ANOVA)** button to check the homogeneity of variances.

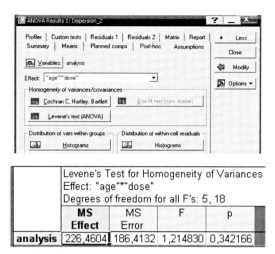

	Levene's Test for Homogeneity of Variances Effect: "age"*"dose" Degrees of freedom for all F's: 5, 18			
	MS **Effect**	MS Error	F	p
analysis	226,4604	186,4132	1,214830	0,342166

After the homogeneity of variances has been checked (*p*=0.342166, that is >0.05), close the ***Levene's test*** window and display the histogram of distribution analysis for all groups as well as the residuals histogram. The visual analysis gives ground to assume that there is insignificant variable abnormality. Close the window.

7. Click the ***Less*** button in the extended ***ANOVA Results*** window. The number of options will be reduced. Press ***All effects/Graphs*** in the ***ANOVA Results*** window. The level of significance equals 0.05 by default.

The table with the variance analysis results will be displayed. According to the values of the significance level, it can be concluded that the null hypothesis is rejected and the alternative one which states that ***age*** (*p*=0.027) and ***dose*** (*p*=0.033) influence the examined analysis is accepted. The common effect of two factors is statistically insignificant. (*p*=0.992).

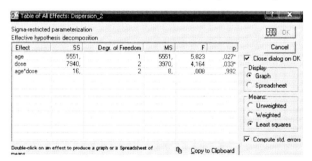

8. Click any parameter in the ***Effect*** section twice for visual analysis and display the graphs where the mean values of the analysis are connected by a jogged line. For instance, the following graph will be displayed by clicking twice on the word ***age***.

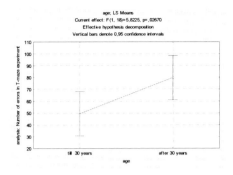

age; LS Means
Current effect: F(1, 18)=5,8225, p=,02670
Effective hypothesis decomposition
Vertical bars denote 0,95 confidence intervals

It indicates that the mean values of the analysis increase with age. Close the graphs.Press the *More results* button and the *Post-hoc* tab in the *ANOVA Results* window to obtain posterior probabilities. Carry out a posterior comparison of groups with different variables analogous to the above example using the *Bonferroni* and *Fisher LSD tests.* Compare the results. Make conclusions.

	Bonferroni test; variable analysis (Dispersion_2 Probabilities for Post Hoc Tests Error: Between MS = 953,38, df = 18,000			
Cell No.	dose	{1} 39,375	{2} 73,000	{3} 81,500
1	level 1		0,128839	0,041362
2	level 2	0,128839		1,000000
3	level 3	0,041362	1,000000	

	LSD test; variable analysis (Dispersion_2) Probabilities for Post Hoc Tests Error: Between MS = 953,38, df = 18,000			
Cell No.	dose	{1} 39,375	{2} 73,000	{3} 81,500
1	level 1		0,042946	0,013787
2	level 2	0,042946		0,588693
3	level 3	0,013787	0,588693	

5.1.11. DIFFERENCES BETWEEN SEVERAL UNRELATED GROUPS. NONPARAMETRIC KRUSKAL-WALLIS H TEST

Nonparametric analogue of Fisher's exact test for ANOVA is the Kruskal-Wallis test. It represents the generalization of the Mann-Whitney test for the case when more than two independent samples are considered. It is also based on the general rank order of values of all samples and does not require the assumption on normality of distribution.

Each value, regardless of what kind of sample it belongs to, and the number of place in the united ordered series - rank R-is given. Then all the individual values are returned to their original samples, and the sums of ranks are calculated individually for each sample. If the differences between the samples are random, the sums of ranks will not differ significantly because the high and low ranks will be equally distributed between the samples. However, if in some samples the low values of ranks dominate; in some samples- high or mean values, the Kruskal-Wallis test will determine these differences. The formula is as follows:

$$H = \frac{12}{N(N+1)} \sum n_m (\overline{R}_m - \overline{R})^2 ,$$

where m – number of compared groups, $\overline{R}_m$ – mean rank in every group, $\overline{R}$ - overall mean rank, $N=n_1+n_2+n_3+...$ ...- total number of observations.

The statistical hypotheses are formulated as follows.

The null hypothesis H_0: there are only random differences between samples 1, 2, 3.

The alternative hypothesis H_1: there are nonrandom differences for the studied feature between samples 1, 2, 3.

If $H_{calc} \geq H_{crit}$, the alternative hypothesis is accepted with a given level of significance or, in other words, if the level of significance is below the critical value, the alternative hypothesis is admitted.

Example 5.6. [6] Influence of oral contraceptives on caffeine elimination

Pregnant women should not drink a lot of strong coffee since it effects on the fetus, and elimination of caffeine is slow during pregnancy. There is a supposition that such a slow elimination of caffeine is observed due to the high level of sex hormones during pregnancy. R. Patwardhan et al. decided to indirectly confirm this hypothesis by determining the rate of caffeine elimination during the period when women are taking contraceptives (because their level of hormones is higher identically to pregnant women). Since the elimination rate is not constant, then the period of half-elimination $T_{1/2}$ is measured. Women taking and not taking contraceptives as well as men took part in the experiment.

Let's make statistical hypotheses.

The null hypothesis H_0: only random differences in time of caffeine elimination exist between the samples.

The alternative hypothesis H_1: nonrandom differences in time of caffeine elimination exist between the samples.

Table 5-6

Men		Women			
		Taking contraceptives		Not taking contraceptives	
$T_{1/2}$	Rank	$T_{1/2}$	Rank	$T_{1/2}$	Rank
2.04	1	5.30	12	10.36	25
5.16	10	7.28	19	13.28	29
6.11	15	8.98	21	11.81	28
5.82	14	6.59	16	4.54	6
5.41	13	4.59	8	11.04	26
3.51	4	5.17	11	10.08	24
3.18	2	7.25	18	14.47	31
4.57	7	3.47	3	9.43	23
4.83	9	7.60	20	13.41	30
11.34	27				
3.79	5				
9.03	22				
7.21	17				

Work order
1. Start *Statistica.*
2. Set variables and name them as *Period* and *Groups.*

1 period	2 groups
2,04	men
5,16	men
6,11	men
5,82	men
5,41	men
3,51	men
3,18	men
4,57	men
4,83	men
11,34	men
3,79	men
9,03	men
7,21	men
5,3	women 1
7,28	women 1
8,98	women 1
6,59	women 1
4,59	women 1
5,17	women 1
7,25	women 1
3,47	women 1
7,6	women 1
10,36	women 2
13,28	women 2
11,81	women 2
4,54	women 2
11,04	women 2
10,08	women 2
14,47	women 2
9,43	women 2
13,41	women 2

3. Choose *Statistics – Nonparametrics*. Select *Comparing multiple indep. samples (groups)*. Press *OK*.

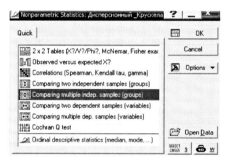

4. In the window *Kruskal-Wallis ANOVA and Median test* press *Variables*.

5. Set *Dependent variable list –period, Indep. (grouping) variable – groups*. Press *OK*.

6. In the window *Kruskal-Wallis ANOVA and Median test* press *Summary: Kruskal-Wallis ANOVA & Median test*.

The window with analyzed data will be opened. The program calculates two tables: *Kruskal-Wallis ANOVA by Ranks* and *Median test*. We are interested only in results of *Kruskal-Wallis ANOVA by Ranks*.

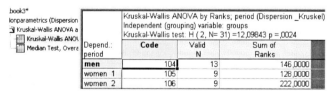

The calculations are displayed in a few lines, the number of which equals the number of independent variables. The greater the sum of the ranks (*Sum of Ranks*) of the group is, the higher the value of this group due to this dependent variable is. It is seen that women of the second group are significantly different from both the first group of women and men on the period of half-elimination. The difference in this case is obvious since the significance level is 0.0024 with the value of H equals 12.094, which is below the critical level and allows accepting the alternative hypothesis. So, there is a relation between the hormone level and half-elimination of caffeine.

If you close the analysis table and display the range chart by clicking **Box & whisker**, it will be seen that the greatest difference is observed in the second group of women compared to men and women of the first group.

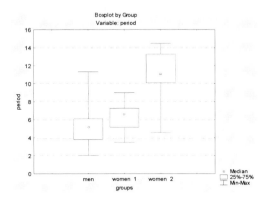

7.   Select the table **Median test.** This method is based on the fact the overall median is calculated for all independent samples, and then it is calculated how many measured values are below and above the median. This leads to the construction of a field table containing $2 \times k$ fields, which is subjected to the **Chi-square test**. As it has been already indicated, the effectiveness of this test is not very high. Close the window.

Note. If there is a difference between several groups, it is necessary to find out what the difference is. To do this it is needed to hold the pairwise (multiple) comparison, in the same way as in the case of the parametric criteria. The Newman-Keuls and Dunnett tests can be used for this purpose. If the samples' sizes are different, the Dunn test is applied.

Conducting pairwise comparisons
1. Consider the same example, but the samples are of the same size with 9 values in each. To do this, remove four last cases for men. Repeat the steps for the previous task.
2. Follow the Kruskal-Wallis test. Its results will vary slightly, but the differences between the groups will be still valid. Close the window.

Workbook1* - Kruskal-Wallis ANOVA by Ranks; period (kruskal_2)				
Workbook1* Nonparametrics (Kruskal_2) Kruskal-Wallis ANOVA a Kruskal-Wallis ANOV Median Test, Overa		Kruskal-Wallis ANOVA by Ranks; period (Kruskal_2) Independent (grouping) variable: groups Kruskal-Wallis test: H (2, N= 27) =13,82363 p =,0010		
	Depend.: period	Code	Valid N	Sum of Ranks
	men	104	9	69,0000
	women 1	105	9	116,0000
	women 2	106	9	193,0000

3. For pairwise comparisons select **Statistics – Basic Statistics/Tables – Breakdown & one-way ANOVA**. Press **OK**.
4. In the window **Statistics by Groups (Breakdown)** press **Variables** and choose the dependent variable **period** in the new window and independent variable (grouping) –**groups.** Press **OK**. Turning back to the window **Statistics by Groups (Breakdown)**, press **OK**.

87

5. In the new window select **Post-hoc**, press the button **Newman-Keuls test & critical ranges**.

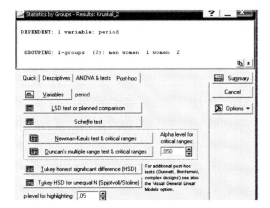

Two tables of analysis will appear, choose the table **Newman-Keuls test**, it will look like:

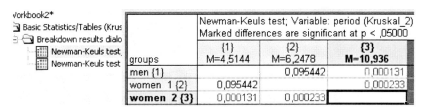

	Newman-Keuls test; Variable: period (Kruskal_2) Marked differences are significant at p < ,05000		
groups	{1} M=4,5144	{2} M=6,2478	{3} M=10,936
men {1}		0,095442	0,000131
women 1 {2}	0,095442		0,000233
women 2 {3}	0,000131	0,000233	

The program highlights in red the significance levels less than 0.05. Thus, the differences between men and the second group of women and between groups of women are statistically significant.

5.1.12. COMPARISON OF SEVERAL DEPENDENT GROUPS (REPEATED MEASURES). FRIEDMAN RANK ANALYSIS OF VARIANCE

If the same group is subjected to several treatments, or simply is observed at different times, the analysis of variance of repeated measurements is applied. If you are not sure that your data are subjected to normal distribution, it is necessary to apply Friedman's non-parametric repeated measures analysis, i.e. the analogue of the parametric analysis of variance of repeated measurements. The Friedman test is similar to the Kruskal-Wallis test. It is based on the rank sequences, which are constructed for all the variables involved in the test. Conditions of applicability: the analyzed characteristics must be quantitative.

Using the Friedman test the null hypothesis that the different treatment methods give almost identical results can be checked. The logic is very simple. Each patient is once subjected to each treatment (or he/she is observed at fixed times). The results of observations of each patient are ordered. The ranks of each line range from 1 to m - the number of the compared treatments. As values for each patient are ordered regardless of all the rest, the number of ranks equals the number of patients involved in the research. Then the sum of ranks is calculated for each treatment method. If the scatter is large, the differences are significant. In order to find the statistical significance the statistics χ^2 is calculated.

$$\chi_r^2 = [\frac{12}{n \cdot m(m+1)} \sum R_i^2] - 3n(m+1)$$

where m – number of conditions (repeated measurements); n – number of tested patients; R_i – sums of ranks for every patient.

If the calculated value χ^2_{calc} does not exceed χ^2_{crit} (for the chosen level of significance p and the corresponding number of degrees of freedom), the null hypothesis of no difference should be accepted. In this case, it can be argued that the signs are derived from a general population. If the calculated value exceeds the critical value (for the chosen level of significance p and the corresponding number of degrees of freedom), the alternative hypothesis on the existence of differences should be accepted. In other words, if $p \leq 0.05$, then the alternative hypothesis is true. In this case, it can be argued that the features are derived from different general populations. This test can be applied in case when homogeneous groups are compared instead of individual patients (randomized block study of the research).

Note. *After the Friedman test it is recommended to conduct pairwise comparisons using the Wilcoxon test and Bonferroni correction.*

Example 5.7. [6] Passive smoking and exercise tolerance

It is a well-known fact that smoking is harmful to patients with coronary artery disease. There are several reasons. First, the heart receives less oxygen, and blood flow worsens. Second, carbon monoxide entering blood binds to hemoglobin displacing oxygen. Third, nicotine reduces myocardial contractility. As a result, tolerance of contractile stress reduces. Does a passive smoking have the same effect? W.S. Aronov tried to answer this question. The experiment involved 10 patients with coronary artery disease. Each patient's exercise capacity was defined as the time of stenocardia attack while working on the exercise bicycle. Then, every tested person had a rest within two hours in a private room, where there were smokers. They either never smoked or smoked 5 cigarettes. In the latter case, the room was ventilated or not. After that the exercise was repeated. The research lasted within three days, and each patient randomly experienced all three types of recreation (one per day) (Table 5-7).

Put forward the statistical hypotheses.

The null hypothesis H_0: only random differences in terms of the exercise capacity exist between samples;

The alternative hypothesis H_1: nonrandom differences exist between samples in terms of the investigated feature, thus, passive smoking affects the exercise tolerance.

Table 5-7

Exercise tolerance in different conditions

patient	Fresh air				Passive smoking, ventilation				Passive smoking without ventilation			
	before		after		before		after		before		after	
	time	rank	time	rank	time	rank	time	rank	time	rank	time	rank
1	193	4	217	6	191	3	149	2	202	5	127	1
2	206	5	214	6	203	4	169	2	189	3	130	1
3	188	4	197	6	181	3	145	2	192	5	128	1
4	375	3	412	6	400	5	306	2	387	4	230	1
5	204	5	199	4	211	6	170	2	196	3	132	1
6	287	3	310	5	304	4	243	2	312	6	198	1
7	221	5	215	4	213	3	158	2	232	6	135	1
8	216	5	223	6	207	3	155	2	209	4	124	1
9	185	4	208	6	186	3	144	2	200	5	129	1
10	231	6	224	4	227	5	172	2	218	3	125	1
Sum of ranks		44		53		39		20		44		10

Work order

1. Start *Statistica.*
2. Enter the 6 columns of values marking them for short as the figure shows.

1 time 1	2 time 1_2	3 time 2	4 time 2_2	5 time 3	6 time 3_2
193	217	191	149	202	127
206	214	203	169	189	130
188	197	181	145	192	128
375	412	400	306	387	230
204	199	211	170	196	132
287	310	304	243	312	198
221	215	213	158	232	135
216	223	207	155	209	124
185	208	186	144	200	129
231	224	227	172	218	125

3. In the operating menu click *Statistics – Nonparametrics*. Choose *Comparing multiple dep. samples (variables)*. Press *OK.*

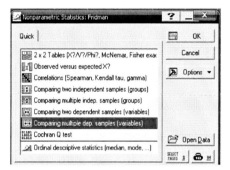

4. Select all six variables pressing *Variables.* Press *OK.* In the new window press the button *Summary: Friedman ANOVA & Kendall's concordance.*

	Friedman ANOVA and Kendall Coeff. of Concordance (Fridman) ANOVA Chi Sqr. (N = 10, df = 5) = 38,40000 p = ,00000 Coeff. of Concordance = ,76800 Aver. rank r = ,74222			
Variable	**Average** **Rank**	Sum of Ranks	Mean	Std.Dev.
time 1	4,300000	43,00000	230,6000	58,65000
time 1_2	5,300000	53,00000	241,9000	67,80438
time 2	4,000000	40,00000	232,3000	68,39274
time 2_2	2,000000	20,00000	181,1000	52,39688
time 3	4,400000	44,00000	233,7000	64,79892
time 3_2	1,000000	10,00000	145,8000	36,86552

5. The table shows that χ^2 *(N=10, cc=5)/Chi Sqr.* χ^2_r *(N = 10, df = 5)* = 38.40000, *p*<0.00000. Thus, the alternative hypothesis is accepted that the differences are statistically significant. The general conclusion: passive smoking reduces the exercise tolerance.

As always, when the differences between several methods of treatment are found, it is necessary to understand what these differences are, i.e. pairwise comparisons of treatments is needed. Since the number of patients is the same, we can use *the Newman-Keuls test.*

5.2. COMPARISON OF THE GROUP BY THE QUALITATIVE ATTRIBUTE

5.2.1. ANALYSIS OF QUALITATIVE ATTRIBUTES WITH FREQUENCY TABLES AND CHI-SQUARE TEST

Very often there are the situations when different groups of observations or values of variables with qualitative features relating to the nominal scale are compared. In this case the frequency tables are constructed.

The term is used to describe the frequency of occurrence. The frequency table is the way to summarize the data set. For each possible value it is indicated how many time it appears in the sample, i.e. actually the table of occurrence is constructed. Sometimes the percent of occurrence (relative frequency) is added to the table. In our example the frequency is still the number of observations in the sample.

Frequency table is used for discrete, nominal and rank data. Of course, it can be used for continuous data, if they are divided into groups.

If there is a matrix of dichotomous variables, coded as 0 and 1, then it is possible to quickly calculate the frequency of ones and zeros for each variable after putting them in the cells. Consider the example.

Example 5.8. Frequency tables for dichotomous feature

Table 5-8

Data in the dichotomous scale

Var 1	Var 2	Var 3	Var 4	Var 5	Var 6	Var 7	Var 8
0	0	1	1	1	1	1	0
0	0	0	0	0	0	0	1
0	1	0	1	0	0	0	0
0	0	0	0	0	0	0	0
0	0	0	1	0	0	1	0
1	1	0	1	0	1	0	0
0	1	0	1	0	0	0	0
0	0	0	1	0	1	0	1
0	0	0	1	0	1	0	0
0	0	0	1	0	1	0	0
0	0	1	0	0	0	0	1
0	0	0	1	0	0	1	0

For the analysis it is necessary to calculate the frequency 0 and 1, or the percents. It's pretty easy to do with the package Statistica.

Work order
1. Start *Statistica.*
2. Enter the matrix of input data. Choose *Basic Statistics/Tables.*
3. In the new window select *Frequency Tables*. Press *OK.*

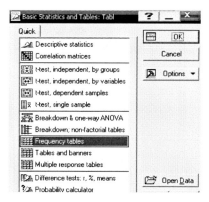

4. In the new window press **Options** and set the option **Percentages (relative frequencies)**. Press the button **Variables** and set 8 variables. Remove the option **Count and report missing data (MD)**. Press **Summary**.

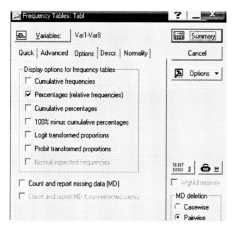

The final table will be constructed which reflects the number of zeros and ones for each of eight variables, as well as the percents. Clicking to the left of the output window, it is possible to get information on each of them.

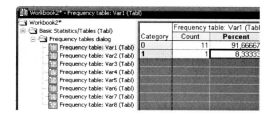

This information can be used for further analysis.

To analyze the frequency table, as a rule, the test χ^2 (or its variants) can be used which was developed by K. Pearson to compare the expected and observed frequencies.

5.2.2. Comparison of ONE group with the population.

COMPARISON OF THE SAMPLE RELATIVE FREQUENCY WITH THE POPULATION
FREQUENCY

Let there be given the sample of n patients. The feature which is interesting for us has the proportion p_d. It is needed to know whether the proportion in the sample differs from the true proportion in the population. Different approaches can be used for this purpose: to calculate χ^2 or Z-test (test of the normal distribution), or to construct a confidence interval. χ^2 will be considered in the following examples. Consider use of the Z-test and confidence interval. Let's suggest the statistical hypotheses.

The null hypothesis H_0 is that the relative frequency of the feature in the sample equals the relative frequency in the population $p_d = p_p$. The alternative H_1 is that the relative frequency in the sample is not equal to the relative frequency in the population $p_d \neq p_p$.

It is necessary to calculate the Z-test with Yates' correction.

$$Z = \frac{|p_p - p_d| - \frac{1}{2n}}{\overline{S}p_d},$$

where p_d— proportion in the group, p_p– relative frequency in the population.

The standard error for the expected population values in the sample is calculated by the formula:

$$\overline{S}p_d = \sqrt{\frac{p_d(1 - p_d)}{n}}$$

If the value $Z_{calc} \geq Z_{crit,}$ then the null hypothesis that the prevalence of the feature in the population equals p_d with the given level of significance is rejected. Otherwise, the null hypothesis is accepted. The limits of the confidence interval can be found using the formula:

$$p_d \pm \overline{S}p_d \cdot z$$

If the value of proportion p_p is known, and if the confidence interval does not include this value, it is possible to assume that for the given level of significance the sample is significantly different from the total population.

Note. *Z-test is determined by the module **Probability calculator** in the software package Statistica. Note that the application of Z-test is valid with the observance of the condition that each value np_d and $n(1 - p_d)$ is more than 5.*

It is possible to calculate the observed and expected frequencies for the known relative frequencies (in the group and the population), and apply χ^2, as in Example 5.10.

Example 5.9. Comparison of preferences in the treatment in the sample and population

40 people were involved in the study of a new drug in the randomized blind test. Some people were treated with the new drug; others were given the old one. Patients were interviewed whether they have preferences of the methods of treatment. It turned out that 30 of them expressed their preferences, and 25 patients preferred the new drug. Were the proportions of patients who prefer these two drugs the same?

Let's formulate the statistical hypotheses.

The null hypothesis H_0: the relative frequency in the population of patients who prefer a new drug is 0.5.

The alternative hypothesis H_1: the relative frequency of patients who prefer a new drug in the population is not equal to 0.5.

Note. *Please note that the sample size decreased to 30 people, but it is more than 10. If the sample size is less than 10, this test cannot be applied.*

93

$$Z = \frac{\left| \frac{25}{30} - 0,5 \right| - \frac{1}{2 \cdot 30}}{\sqrt{\frac{\frac{25}{30} \cdot (1 - \frac{25}{30})}{30}}} \approx 0.313/0.06 \approx 5.21$$

Then it is necessary to apply the Table of the Laplace transforms function. If the value $Z \geq Z_{crit}$ for the given level of significance, then the alternative hypothesis is accepted, and the null hypothesis is rejected that these two drugs are preferred equally often.

You can also use the module *Probability calculator*. To do this choose *Statistics - Basic Statistics / Tables - Probability calculator* in the operating menu. If the sample is large (n> 30), then select the type of distribution *Z(*Normal*)*, of Z, and set the option: *Inwerse* - inverse distribution function; *Two-tailed, 1-Cumulative p; mean-0;* standard deviation - *st.dev-1*, set the level of significance *p = 0.05*. Click *Compute*. The *Z value* will be calculated. For the given probability it is approximately 1.96.

If the sample is small but not less than 10, then use the distribution *t(Student)*. Set the same options, but also keep a number of degrees of freedom *df=n-1=29*. T_{crit}=2.04. Since $Z > t_{crit}$, the alternative hypothesis is true that these two drugs are preferred in the population with varying frequency.

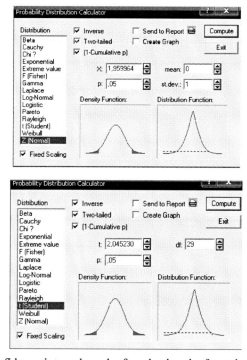

The limits of the confidence interval can be found using the formula:

$$p_d \pm \overline{S}p_d \cdot z$$

If the confidence interval does not include the value of the population 0.5, we can assume that for the given level of significance the sample is significantly different from the total population.

94

5.2.3. COMPARISON OF OBSERVED AND EXPECTED FREQUENCIES IN THE TWO GROUPS USING CHI-SQUARE

Example 5.10. The prevalence of the disease in some groups
Let it be known that the prevalence of certain diseases in groups is presented by the following data

Table 5-9

	Observed frequencies	Expected frequencies
1 group	55	31
2 group	170	185

Let's assume the statistical hypotheses.
The null hypothesis H_0: observed and expected frequencies are equal.
The alternative hypothesis H_1: the observed and expected frequencies are not equal. χ^2 includes the observed frequencies O and the expected frequencies E.

$$\chi^2 = \sum \frac{\left(|O-E|-\frac{1}{2}\right)^2}{E}$$

Work order
1. Set the data in *Statistica*. In the operational menu select *Statistics –Nonparametrics - Observed versus expected X*. Press *OK*.

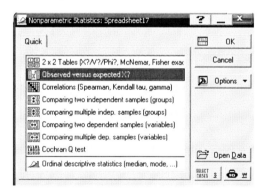

2. In the window *Observed vs. Expected Frequency* press the button *Variables* and select the variables. Press *OK*. Turning back to the first window press *Summary*.
The table of analysis will be displayed. At the top the specified level of significance is indicated. In the right column at the bottom χ^2 is shown. It is indicated in the headline of the table.

Case	observed observed	expected expected	O - E	(O-E)**2 /E
C: 1	55,0000	31,0000	24,0000	18,58065
C: 2	170,0000	185,0000	-15,0000	1,21622
Sum	225,0000	216,0000	9,0000	19,79686

Observed vs. Expected Frequencies (Spreadsheet17)
Chi-Square = 19,79686 df = 1 p < ,000009
NOTE: Unequal sums of obs. & exp. frequencies

If $p \geq 0.05$, the null hypothesis of no difference between observed and expected frequencies for the studied feature should be accepted.

If $p < 0.05$, the alternative hypothesis that the differences between the observed and expected frequencies exist should be accepted. In our case, $p < 0.000009$, so the alternative hypothesis is accepted.

Note. *Remember that when using any version of χ^2, make sure that none of the expected frequencies was less than 5. Otherwise the results will be biased. If one of the expected frequencies is less than 5, the Fisher's exact test should be applied.*

Example 5.11. Seasonality of infectious diseases

Let's say that some infectious diseases prevalent in some areas in different months. The frequencies of distribution will be called observed. It is necessary to determine whether the nature of the disease is seasonal. In other words, whether the frequencies are distributed equally by months.

Before proceeding to the statistical analysis, we formulate the statistical hypotheses.

The null hypothesis H_0: the expected frequencies (sum of diseased for the year divided by 12 months) equal the observed frequencies (the observed frequencies of diseased by months).

The alternative hypothesis (H_1): the observed frequencies differ from the expected, and studied disease is seasonal.

Work order

1. Start **Statistica**. In the window **Add cases** set the number of added lines (2). Press **OK**.

2. Indicate the columns. Instead of **Var1** in the line **Name** enter **Observed**, and instead of **Var2 –expected**. Press **OK**.

3. Enter the names of months. For this purpose make a double-click on the number of each line. Enter the values of variables. Type 77.75 for all expected frequencies (the amount of diseased per year is 993. It is divided by 12, and we obtain 77.75). The table will look like this:

	1 observed	2 expected
January	125	77,75
February	150	77,75
March	80	77,75
April	50	77,75
May	40	77,75
June	43	77,75
July	80	77,75
August	75	77,75
September	80	77,75
October	65	77,75
November	50	77,75
December	95	77,75

4. In the operational menu select **Statistics – Nonparametrics -Observed versus expected X?** (see Example 5.10). Press **OK**.

5. Click **Variables** in the appeared window. Select **Expected** and **O**bserved for different frequencies. Press **OK**. Click **Summary** in the previous window.

6. The table of results shows that the statistics subject to the distribution **Chi-Square** (χ^2=194.9904) was used; the number of degrees of freedom is 11 (**cc/df = 11**), and the probability of the null hypothesis is less than 0.001 ($p < 0.000000$), which considerably less than the critical significance level 0.05. This means that the null hypothesis is rejected, and the alternative one is accepted.

Case	Observed vs. Expected Frequencies (Infektion) Chi-Square = 155,7331 df = 11 p < 0,000000			
	observed observed	expected expected	O - E	(O-E)**2 /E
January	125,0000	77,7500	47,2500	28,7146
February	150,0000	77,7500	72,2500	67,1391
March	80,0000	77,7500	2,2500	0,0651
April	50,0000	77,7500	-27,7500	9,9043
May	40,0000	77,7500	-37,7500	18,3288
June	43,0000	77,7500	-34,7500	15,5314
July	80,0000	77,7500	2,2500	0,0651
August	75,0000	77,7500	-2,7500	0,0973
September	80,0000	77,7500	2,2500	0,0651
October	65,0000	77,7500	-12,7500	2,0908
November	50,0000	77,7500	-27,7500	9,9043
December	95,0000	77,7500	17,2500	3,8272
Sum	933,0000	933,0000	0,0000	155,7331

Thus, we have found that the studied disease is seasonal.

5.2.4. CONSTRUCTION OF A CROSSTABULATION TABLE. COMPARISON OF FREQUENCIES IN TWO GROUPS BY FISHER'S EXACT TEST

Example 5.12. Study of the effectiveness of vaccinations
Suppose you want to explore the connection between vaccination against certain diseases and the disease incidence. Suppose you have the following data:

Table 5-10

Patient	Sex	Year of birth	Inoculation	Disease
Abramov A.A	M	1945	no	yes
Ivanov I.N.	M	1956	yes	no
Smirnov I.I.	M	1983	yes	yes
Sidorov K.K.	M	1976	yes	yes
Bobrov S. N	M	1967	no	yes
Kozlov S.M.	M	1977	yes	no
Oparina M.T.	w	1964	no	no
Rebrov A.A.	M	1988	no	no
Kovrov K.T.	M	1975	yes	yes
Mironov P.G.	M	1959	yes	no

The studied variables **Inoculation** and **Disease** are categorical and dichotomous as they take only two values: yes or no. The patient falls into one of two categories. It is necessary to construct the **Crosstabulation Table** to analyze the data. There are tables of various size n × n. The simplest is the 2 × 2 table (fourfold table). In this example it will be constructed because it has only 4 combinations (yes, yes), (yes, no), (no, no), (no, yes) of variables **Inoculation** and **Disease**.

Initial data for the analysis

	1 inoculation	2 disease
Abramov A.A	no	yes
Ivanov I.N.	yes	no
Smirnov I.I.	yes	yes
Sidorov K.K.	yes	yes
Bobrov S. N	no	yes
Kozlov S.M.	yes	no
Oparina M.T.	no	no
Rebrov A.A.	yes	no
Kovrov K.T.	no	yes
Mironov P.G.	yes	no

Let's formulate the statistical hypotheses.

The null hypothesis H_0: there is no relationship between the vaccination and the number diseased.

The alternative hypothesis H_1: there is a relationship between the vaccination and the number of diseased.

In other words, the frequency of diseased from the group without vaccination is greater than the frequency of diseased from the group with vaccination, or the frequency of diseased in the group without vaccination is greater than the frequency of diseased in the group with vaccination. Note that only unilateral alternative is considered; deviation - only to the higher side.

Work order

1. Start *Statistica.* Enter the data from the initial table. Identify the first variable as *Inoculation,* the second one *-Diseases*

2. Select *Statistics – Basic Statistics/Tables*. Press *Tables and banners.* Press *OK.*

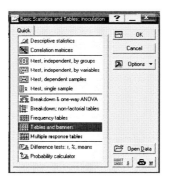

3. In the dialog box *Crosstabulation Tables* select the tab *Stub-and-Banner*, set the toggle button in the position *Use selected grouping codes only,* press the button *Specify Tables (select Variables)*.

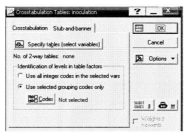

4. Choose the variables. *First variable list –Inoculation,* and *Second variable list – Diseases.*

You can only choose several grouping variables (i.e. variables that define the division of the patients into groups), for us it is sufficient to select only two variables. Click *OK* and return to the dialog box of setting the table, where you should click *Codes*. In the new window, where codes are given for grouping factors, click *All*. Click *OK*. The variables will be coded as 1 and 0 automatically.

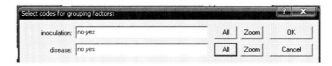

5.   In the window ***Crosstabulation Tables*** press ***OK.*** In the opened window ***Crosstabulation Tables Results*** select ***Options*** and set the options of needed tests (Pearson, Fisher etc), and also set the percents if you need to know the percents for every cell.

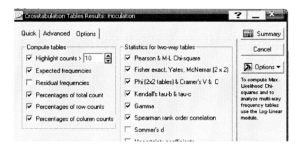

6.   Press ***Advanced*** and the button ***Detailed two-way Tables.***

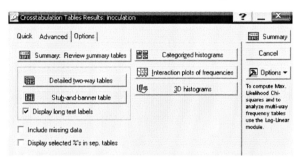

There will be three tables of analysis. Select the table ***2-Way Summary Table: Observed Frequencies***. It contains the observed frequencies and percentages by lines and columns, and the total percents. Looking at the table you see, for example, that one person from studied people had no vaccinations, and did not get sick; 3 people had vaccinations and got sick; 4 people were vaccinated and did not get sick; 2 persons were vaccinated and got sick.

The bottom line (**Totals**) shows the sum of values in the columns. In the right column there is the sum of values in the lines. These values are sometimes called marginal or boundary since they are on the edges of the table.

kbook22*			
Basic Statistics/Tables (inoculation)		2-Way Summary Table: Observed Frequencie	
Crosstabulation results dialog		Marked cells have counts > 10	
2-Way Summary Table: Observed Frequencies (ino		disease	disease	Row
2-Way Summary Table: Expected Frequencies (inoc	inoculation	no	yes	Totals
Statistics: inoculation(2) x disease(2) (inoculation)	**no**	1	3	4
	Column %	20,00%	60,00%	
	Row %	25,00%	75,00%	
	Total %	10,00%	30,00%	40,00%
	yes	4	2	6
	Column %	80,00%	40,00%	
	Row %	66,67%	33,33%	
	Total %	40,00%	20,00%	60,00%
	Totals	5	5	10
	Total %	50,00%	50,00%	100,00%

Select the table ***2-Way Summary Table: Expected Frequencies***. They are needed for the choice of the test.

Note. *There are well-known recommendations of Kochran for 2×2 tables: if the sum of all the frequencies in the table is less than 20, the Fisher exact test should be used. If the sum of* *the frequencies is greater than 40, then we can apply χ^2 with continuity correction. However, these recommendations are not universal.*

As in the table *2-Way Summary Table: Expected Frequencies* the frequency is less than 4 in one of the cells, which is less than 5, then the Fisher's test should be selected to analyze the difference between the frequencies and information allowing estimating the relationship between categorical variables *Inoculation* and *Diseases*.

Workbook22* - 2-Way Summary Table: Expected Frequencies (inoculation)			

Workbook22*
- Basic Statistics/Tables (inoculation)
- Crosstabulation results dialog
  - 2-Way Summary Table: Observed Frequencies (ino
  - 2-Way Summary Table: Expected Frequencies (ino
  - Statistics: inoculation(2) x disease(2) (inoculation)

2-Way Summary Table: Expected Frequencies (inoculation) Marked cells have counts > 10			
inoculation	disease no	disease yes	Row Totals
no	2,000000	2,000000	4,00000
yes	3,000000	3,000000	6,00000
Totals	5,000000	5,000000	10,00000

Select the table *Statistics*.

:book22*
- lasic Statistics/Tables (inoculation)
- Crosstabulation results dialog
  - 2-Way Summary Table: Observed Frequencies (ino
  - 2-Way Summary Table: Expected Frequencies (ino
  - Statistics: inoculation(2) x disease(2) (inoculation)

Statistic	Statistics: inoculation(2) x disease(2) (inoculation)		
	Chi-square	df	p
Pearson Chi-square	1,666667	df=1	p=,19671
M-L Chi-square	1,726092	df=1	p=,18891
Yates Chi-square	,4166667	df=1	p=,51861
Fisher exact, one-tailed			p=,26190
two-tailed			p=,52381
McNemar Chi-square (A/D)	0,000000	df=1	p=1,0000
(B/C)	0,000000	df=1	p=1,0000
Phi for 2 x 2 tables	-,408248		
Tetrachoric correlation	-,607073		
Contingency coefficient	,3779645		
Kendall's tau b & c	b=-,408248	c=-,400000	
Gamma	-,714286		
Spearman Rank R	-,408248	t=-1,265	p=,24150

The Fisher's exact test is 0.26 which is much larger than the critical 0.05. Hence, the null hypothesis that the frequency of diseased in the group without vaccination is greater than the frequency of diseased in the group with vaccination is accepted

Please note that the Fisher's exact test and χ^2 with the Yates correction (if it is divided by two because of one-sided hypothesis) have the same value 0.26. And the expected frequency is less than 5 in one of the cells. Thus, the recommendations of Kochran on the conditions of applicability of the tests are not universal.

Now look at the graphical representation of the table.

7.   Turn back to the window *Crosstabulation Tables Results*, choose the tab *Advanced*, press *3D Histograms*. As a result, the 3D plot will be displayed. Close it.

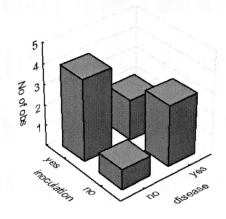

8.   In the dialog box *Crosstabulation Tables Results*, press *Advanced*, press the button *Categorized histograms*, and the following plots will be displayed:

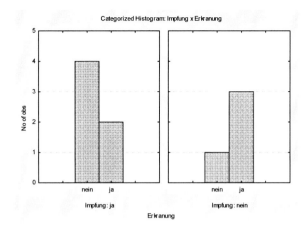

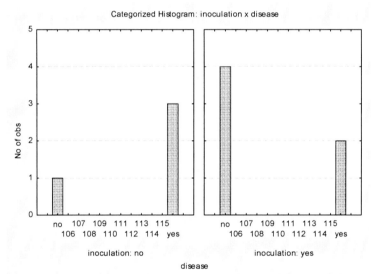

As you can see, in the categorical plot all the examinees are divided into two categories: **Inoculation** - no, **Inoculation** - yes. The plot shows that the number of diseased who did not have inoculation is more than the number of diseased in the group of vaccinated people.

If the vaccine was not made, the number of diseased is 3, and the number of not diseased is - 1. If the vaccine was made, the number of not diseased is 4, and the number of diseased is 2. Close the window.

Consider one more plot – the Interaction Plot.

9.   In the dialog box *Crosstabulation Tables Results* press the tab *Advanced*, press the button *Interaction plots of frequencies*. You will see the following plot:

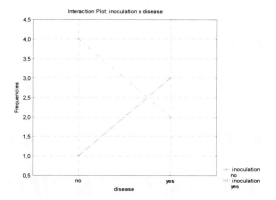

The plot shows that the number of people who were vaccinated but infected is less than the number of people who were not vaccinated and infected. Lines on the plot cross, therefore, the factors are interacting. If the lines are parallel, we will say that there is no interaction between the factors.

So, the plot shows there is the relationship between the factors. However, this difference is not statistically significant. Perhaps with a larger sample size, the significance level would fall below the critical level.

Note. *If there are many variables in the table, it is possible to cross-tabulate up to 30 variables. The figure below shows the crosstabulation of first six variables with the seventh from a certain list of seven variables.*

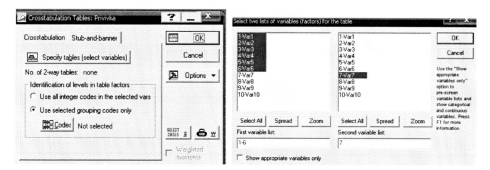

5.2.5. COMPARISON OF FREQUENCIES WITH THE CROSSTABULATION TABLE 2 × 2 IN TWO INDEPENDENT SAMPLES USING THE CHI-SQUARE TEST

Let's take an example how you can find out the significance of differences for cross-tabulated data and draw the conclusion about the dependence or relationship between the features.

Note. *If the tables are made manually, it is necessary to ensure that the indicator A mutually excludes the indicator B (yes/no, exacerbation/remission).*

Example 5.13. [6]. Shunt thrombosis in hemodialysis patients

Hemodialysis can save the lives of people suffering from chronic renal failure. Patient's blood is passed through an artificial kidney - the device, which removes metabolic products from blood. The artificial kidney is connected to the patient's artery and vein; and blood from the artery enters the apparatus, and then -already cleaned, - in the vein. Since dialysis is carried out regularly, the patient is set the arteriovenous shunt. The Teflon tubes are placed in the artery and vein in the forearm, their ends are output and connected with each other. With the procedure tubes are disconnected and attached to the device. The contact with the foreign surface and turbulence of blood flow often lead to the thrombosis in the shunt. Clots of blood have to be removed regularly, and in severe cases even the shunt is changed. Guided by the fact that aspirin prevents the formation of blood clots, H.R. Harter and colleagues decided to check if it is possible to reduce the risk of thrombosis with the prescription of small doses of aspirin (160 mg / day) in 1979.

All patients who agreed to participate in the test and did not have contraindications to aspirin were randomly divided into two groups: the 1st received placebo, 2nd - aspirin. Neither the doctor who gave the drug, nor the patient knew whether it was aspirin or not. Such a method of testing (it is called a double blind) excludes favoring by the doctor or the patient and provides with the most reliable results. Groups did not differ in age, sex and duration of hemodialysis.

The shunt thrombosis occurred in 18 of 25 cases in the first group. 6 patients out of 19 had the shunt thrombosis in the second group. The total number of patients was 44. Can we speak of a statistically significant difference in the proportion of patients with thrombosis, and thus the effectiveness of aspirin?

Let's put forward the statistical hypotheses.

The null hypothesis H_0: frequencies of the shunt thrombosis are the same in the groups with application of placebo and aspirin.

The alternative hypothesis H_1: frequencies of the shunt thrombosis in the groups with placebo and aspirin are different.

To select a statistical test we should note that the two samples are independent; they are made up of patients treated with aspirin, and patients treated with placebo. The data are presented by the frequency table; the total sum of frequencies is 44. Therefore, taking into account the recommendations of Kochran for 2×2 tables, it is necessary to use χ^2 with Yates corrected Chi-square. Please note that in contrast to the task of vaccination, the data is already crosstabulated. Therefore, it is possible to use another module of the software package Statistica.

Table 5-11

Effect of aspirin on thrombosis: crosstabulation table

	Placebo	Aspirin
Thrombosis: yes	18	6
Thrombosis: no	7	13

Work order

1. Start **Statistica.** In the operational menu choose **Statistics –Nonparametrics**. In the opened window select **2×2 Tables (X?/V?/Phi?, McNemar, Fisher exact)** and press **OK**.

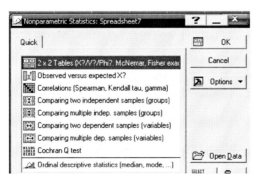

2. The window to fill the table will be opened. Type four values of frequencies. The left column of the window corresponds to the left column of the table 5-11 (placebo), and the right - to the right one (Aspirin). The top line corresponds to the top of the table 5-11 (Thrombosis: yes), and the lowest - to the lowest one (Thrombosis: no). We will see the following:

103

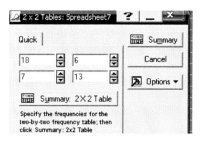

3. Press the button **Summary**. The detailed table with the results of statistical analysis will be displayed:

2 x 2 Table (Spreadsheet7)			
	Column 1	Column 2	Row Totals
Frequencies, row 1	18	6	24
Percent of total	40,909%	13,636%	54,545%
Frequencies, row 2	7	13	20
Percent of total	15,909%	29,545%	45,455%
Column totals	25	19	44
Percent of total	56,818%	43,182%	
Chi-square (df=1)	7,11	p= ,0077	
V-square (df=1)	6,95	p= ,0084	
Yates corrected Chi-square	5,58	p= ,0182	
Phi-square	,16168		
Fisher exact p, one-tailed		p= ,0087	
two-tailed		p= ,0138	
McNemar Chi-square (A/D)	,52	p= ,4725	
Chi-square (B/C)	0,00	p=1,0000	

Let's consider the information in the resulting table. The table shows that patients who took aspirin had thrombosis in 13.6% of cases (6/44), whereas patients treated with placebo, had it more often - in 40.9% (18/44). However, these data are insufficient for the correct conclusion since it is necessary to estimate the statistical significance of the differences with the help of properly selected test.

The table shows that the Yates corrected Chi-square value equals 5.58, and the probability of the null hypothesis $p = 0.0182$. Consequently, we reject it and accept the alternative hypothesis which states that the frequency of thrombosis with aspirin and placebo are different. Thus, we conclude that taking aspirin **statistically significantly** reduced by 27.3% the frequency of thrombosis ($\chi^2 = 5.58$; $p = 0.018$) because of improved rheological properties of blood due to its disaggregant and anticoagulant activity.

5.2.6. COMPARISON OF QUALITATIVE FEATURES (EXPRESSED IN FREQUENCIES) IN 2 INDEPENDENT GROUPS USING THE FISHER'S EXACT TEST

Example 5.14. [6]. Electroanalgesia in dentistry

T. Bishop studied the effectiveness of high-frequency nerve stimulation as an analgesic for tooth extraction in 1986. All patients were connected to the device, but in some cases it worked, and in others was turned off. Neither the dentist nor the patient knew whether the device worked or not. Do the following data of the 2×2 crosstabulation table show that the high-frequency nerve stimulation is an effective analgesic method?

Table 5-12

Electroanalgesia: crosstabulation table

Indicator	Device is turned on	Device is turned off	Total
Pain (yes)	$a=7$	$b=2$	9
Pain (no)	$c=1$	$d=8$	9
Total	8	10	18

Let's put forward the statistical hypotheses.

The null hypothesis H_0: patients experience pain equally often regardless the device (when it is turned on and switched off)

The alternative hypothesis H_1: patients experience pain with different frequencies depending on the condition of the device (when it is turned on and switched off)

Let's analyze the situation to choose the test:
- There are two independent samples;
- Data are presented as categorical (qualitative) variables;
- The total sum of the frequencies is 18, which is less than 20, and there are the expected frequencies less than 5.

Consider how to calculate the expected numbers. 8 patients were treated with the turned on device; 10 patients were treated with the switched off device. Patients feel pain in 9 cases out of 18, i.e. in 50% of cases, and pain did not appear in 9 of 18 cases, i.e. also the percent makes 50%. If we have accepted as the null hypothesis the fact that the device has no effect on the incidence of pain, then calculating how much is 50% of 10 and 8, we will find the expected numbers. The expected numbers for patients with pain when the device is switched off and turned on are 5 and 4 respectively. In the same way we calculate the expected numbers for the patients with no pain. They also make up 50%, but the numbers are 9 and 9. This numbers will be 4.5 and 4.5. Therefore, the Fisher exact test is needed which is presented in two versions – one-tailed and two-tailed.

Choice of the variant depends on the objectives of the research and previously obtained information. Two-tailed version of any test is chosen if you want to check whether there are significant differences. One-tailed version of any test is selected if it is necessary to prove that the factor being studied (in this case, electroanalgesia) improves the outcome. Let's check the null hypothesis using the two-tailed test.

Work order

1. Start the software package *Statistica.* Choose *Statistics –Nonparametrics* in the operational menu.

2. In the opened window choose **2×2 Tables (X?/V?/Phi?, McNemar, Fisher exact)** and press *OK*.

3. Input the value of frequencies according to the table, so that the left column of the window corresponds to the left column of the Table 5-12 (the device is turned on), and the right column corresponds to the right one (the device is switched off.) The following table will be displayed:

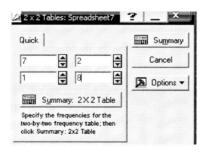

4. Press *OK*. You will see the detailed table with the statistical results.

2 x 2 Table (Spreadsheet7)			
	Column 1	Column 2	Row Totals
Frequencies, row 1	7	2	9
Percent of total	38,889%	11,111%	50,000%
Frequencies, row 2	1	8	9
Percent of total	5,556%	44,444%	50,000%
Column totals	8	10	18
Percent of total	44,444%	55,556%	
Chi-square (df=1)	8,10	p= ,0044	
V-square (df=1)	7,65	p= ,0057	
Yates corrected Chi-square	5,63	p= ,0177	
Phi-square	,45000		
Fisher exact p, one-tailed		p= ,0076	
two-tailed		p= ,0152	
McNemar Chi-square (A/D)	0,00	p=1,0000	
Chi-square (B/C)	0,00	p=1,0000	

The table shows that with the turned on device 38.9% (7/18) of patients did not feel the pain, and with the switched off device 11.1% patients felt the pain (2/18). However, these data are insufficient for the correct conclusion since it is necessary to estimate the statistical significance of the differences with the help of the properly selected test.

The probability of the null hypothesis due to the Fisher exact two-tailed test is $p = 0.0152$ which is significantly lower than 0.05. Since the probability of the null hypothesis is not enough to accept it, we accept the alternative hypothesis, which states that with the switched off device the patients feel pain with different frequencies. Thus, we conclude that use of electroanalgesia significantly (by 27.8%) reduces the pain.

5.2.7. COMPARISON OF QUALITATIVE FEATURES (EXPRESSED IN FREQUENCIES) IN TWO RELATED SAMPLES WITH THE HELP OF MCNEMAR TEST

McNemar test is used only with the dichotomous variables. In this case it is considered whether there are some changes in the structure of their values distribution. In the majority of cases the comparison is made taking into account the time factor due to the scheme "before - after".

Example 5.15. [6]. Rhinitis treatment by vasoconstrictors

Alpha-adrenomimetics are widely used in rhinitis treatment as vasoconstrictors which allow reducing the rhinedema and mucus secretion, thereby restoring the nasal breathing. There are many well-known drugs of this pharmacological group. The children's hospital purchased two of them: spironas and rinolisin.

170 children were observed. The first day each child took only spironas; the second- only rinolisin. After 10 minutes the nasal breathing was estimated. Thus, different methods of treatment were applied to the same groups. The following results were achieved:

Table 5-13

The efficiency of the two vasoconstrictors

Medicine		Spironas	
	Effect	Nasal stuffiness	Clear breathing
Rinolosin	Nasal stuffiness	$a = 33$	$b = 53$
	Clear breathing	$c = 48$	$d = 36$

The table shows that sometimes both drugs helped the patients, and sometimes only one medicine was effective. In some cases none of them helped. So spironas helped 53 patients, and rinolisin was effective in 48 cases. Both drugs helped in 36 cases, and none helped 33 patients. It is needed to find out which drug is more effective. As we estimate the ability of drugs to restore the nasal breathing, and the frequencies of breathing recovery are located in cells b and c, then the probability of the null hypothesis should be determined by the contents of the cells (b/c).

Let's formulate the statistical hypotheses.

The null hypothesis H_0: both products give the same frequencies of recovery of the nasal breathing.

The alternative hypothesis H_1: the frequency of recovery of the nasal breathing is different with two treatment methods.

Since there is only one sample - the group of patients which was initially prescribed one drug, and then on the second day another drug, and that the information is presented in the form of categorical variables - "Nasal stuffiness " and " Clear breathing "- McNemar test should be applied.

Work order

1. Start the software package *Statistica.* Choose the submenu *Statistics – Nonparametrics.*

2. In the opened window select **2×2 Tables (X?/V?/Phi?, McNemar, Fisher exact)** and press *OK*.

3. In tables 2×2 (*note that this is not a crosstabulation table since each object is considered twice*) the following names of cells are applied: *a*-top left, *b* - top right, *c* - lower left and *d* - lower right. The following table will be displayed:

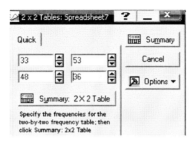

4. Click *Summary*. The table with the statistical results will be displayed:

2 x 2 Table (Spreadsheet7)			
	Column 1	Column 2	Row Totals
Frequencies, row 1	33	53	86
Percent of total	19,412%	31,176%	50,588%
Frequencies, row 2	48	36	84
Percent of total	28,235%	21,176%	49,412%
Column totals	81	89	170
Percent of total	47,647%	52,353%	
Chi-square (df=1)	6,00	p= ,0143	
V-square (df=1)	5,97	p= ,0146	
Yates corrected Chi-square	5,27	p= ,0217	
Phi-square	,03531		
Fisher exact p, one-tailed		p= ,0107	
two-tailed		p= ,0210	
McNemar Chi-square (A/D)	,06	p= ,8097	
Chi-square (B/C)	,16	p= ,6906	

The table shows that spironas helped approximately 31.2% (53/170) patients, rinolisin-28.2% (48/170). However, these data are insufficient for the correct conclusion since it is necessary to estimate the statistical significance of the differences using *McNemar test*.

McNemar test subject to the distribution χ^2 is presented in two versions-*Chi-square (a/d)* and *Chi-square (b/c).* In our case the probability of the null hypothesis should be determined by Chi-square (*b/c*). As the table shows this test is 0.16, and the corresponding probability is 0.69, which is significantly higher than the critical level of significance 0.05. On this basis, we accept the null hypothesis.

Thus, we conclude that there is no statistically significant differences between spironas and rinolisin due to the ability to recover the nasal breathing ($\chi^2 = 0.16$; $p = 0.69$).

It should be emphasized that if we mistakenly used Chi-square test or Fisher exact two-tailed test, the conclusion would be opposite. Since $p = 0.014$ and $p = 0.021$, respectively, we could incorrectly accept the alternative hypothesis on the differential effect of drugs on the nasal breathing.

5.2.8 THE CONSTRUCTION OF THE CONFIDENCE INTERVAL FOR THE DIFFERENCE OF RELATIVE FREQUENCIES IN RELATED SAMPLES (BEFORE AND AFTER TREATMENT)

The difference of the relative frequencies of the binary feature is denoted as follows:

$$\Delta = p_{d1} - p_{d2}$$

The observed relative frequencies with the presence of a particular feature in these two states:

$$p_{d1} = \frac{a+b}{n}, \quad p_{d2} = \frac{a+c}{n}$$

They will be different, if b and c are different. Thus, attention is paid only to the matched pairs.

$$\Delta p = \frac{a+b}{n} - \frac{a+c}{n} = \frac{b-c}{n},$$

where $n = a + b + c + d$ – total number of observations.

It is needed to calculate the standard error for the mean of the relative frequencies difference.

$$\bar{S}_\Delta = \frac{1}{n}\sqrt{b + c - \frac{(b-c)^2}{n}}$$

The limits of the confidence interval: $\Delta p \pm t \cdot \bar{S}_\Delta$

In case of the large sample size and the significance level equals 0.05, the Student's t quantile t = 1.96. As regards the small sample size, indicate the degree of freedom as $k = n - 1$ and the level of significance in the module *Probability calculator*.

If the confidence interval does not contain zero, we can say with a given reliability, for example, 95%, that relative frequencies before and after treatment are different. If the confidence interval includes zero, we can say with a given reliability, for example, 95%, that relative frequencies before and after treatment are not different.

5.2.9. Q KOCHRAN TEST FOR REPEATED TESTS

Q Kochran test is the development of the χ^2 *McNemar test*. It checks whether the difference is significant if several dichotomous variables taking the values 0 or 1 for several related samples are compared. If the variables are not within the nominal scale, they must be made dichotomized.

Example 5.16. Season and mood

Let's suppose we are interested how the season influences the mood of the tested people. Yes - negative, no- positive. The polls were carried out in autumn, winter and summer, and thus it is needed to know whether the results of them have changed over the time.

Table 5-14

Influence of the season on mood

	poll_1(winter)	poll_2 (spring)	poll_3(summer)
1	no	no	no
2	yes	yes	no
3	no	no	no
4	no	no	no
5	yes	yes	no
6	yes	yes	no
7	yes	yes	no
8	no	yes	no
9	yes	no	no
10	no	no	no
11	yes	yes	yes
12	yes	yes	yes
13	yes	yes	no
14	yes	yes	no
15	yes	yes	no
16	yes	yes	yes
17	yes	yes	no
18	yes	yes	no

Let's put forward the statistical hypotheses.

The null hypothesis H_0: there is no difference in mood.

The alternative hypothesis H_1: there is a difference in mood of the respondents in the different seasons.

Work order

1. Start the software package *Statistica*. Input the variables, giving them the values 0 (no) and 1 (yes). Name them *poll_1, poll_2, poll_3.*

2. Choose *Statistics –Nonparametrics* in the operational menu. Select the procedure *Cochran Q test.* Press **OK.**

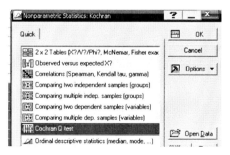

3. Pressing the button *Variables*, choose all the variables. Press *Summary* or the button *Summary: Cochran Q test.*

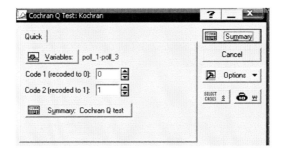

The table with the results of ***Cochran Q test*** will be displayed:

	Cochran Q Test (Kochran) Number of valid cases:18 Q = 18,18182, df = 2, p < ,000113		
Variable	**Sum**	Percent 0's	Percent 1's
poll_1	13,00000	27,77778	72,22222
poll_2	13,00000	27,77778	72,22222
poll_3	3,00000	83,33333	16,66667

The coefficient Q = 18.18, the significance level of *p* is less than 0.000113. This suggests that the groups differ from each other. The rightmost column shows the percentage of "yes" responses (Percent $1's$). The number of respondents with a bad mood in summer (poll_3) decreased. Thus confirmed the alternative hypothesis of differences in mood at different times of the year, indicating the connection of season and mood of the respondents. The histograms can be constructed to illustrate that. For this purpose right-click in the data area and select ***Histograms*** in the drop down menu.

5.2.10. COMPARISON OF 2 QUALITATIVE FEATURES IN TWO INDEPENDENT SAMPLES EXPRESSED AS A PERCENTAGE (COMPARISON OF THE RELATIVE FREQUENCIES WITHIN ONE GROUP AND TWO GROUPS)

It is needed to find out whether two different groups of patients differ according to the feature, the presence of which in both groups is coded by 1, and the absence of which is coded by zero.

Note. *The percents in the group can be calculated with the help of the module **Frequency Tables** as in* **Example 5.8** *of this chapter.*

Example 5.17.[6]. Anesthesia by halothane and morphine

Halothane and morphine have different effect on blood pressure. However, it is more important for the clinicians to know is there any difference in postsurgical mortality. According to the research of T. Conahan et al. in 1973, 16 of 122 patients operated under halothane anesthesia died that constituted 13.1%. As regards anesthesia by morphine, 20 of 134 patients died that makes 14.9%. Lethality was lower by approximately 2% under halothane anesthesia. Is it possible to assume that morphine is more dangerous than halothane, or the result is not regular?

Let's formulate the statistical hypotheses.

The null hypothesis H_0: lethality under anesthesia by halothane and morphine is equal. The alternative hypothesis H_1: lethality under anesthesia by halothane and morphine is different.

Since the samples are independent, their size is more than 100, the data is expressed in percent, Z-test should be used for the proportion.

Work order
1. Start *Statistica*. Select *Basic Statistics/Tables*.
2. Select *Difference tests: r, %, means.* Click *OK.*

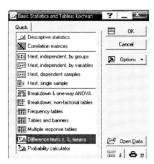

3.   In the *Difference between two proportions* dialogue box select *Pr.* 1: and type (on a keyboard or using a computer mouse) the decimal percentage of lethality in the group under halothane anesthesia. For this purpose divide 13.1% by 100 % and type 0.131. By analogy type 0.149 in the line *Pr.* 2:. Then type the samples size: $N1$ = 122 and $N2$=134. As regards the type of the test, select *Two sided*. Click the *Compute* button.

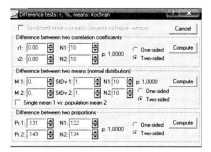

The window of analysis will appear which shows that the probability of the null hypothesis ($p = 0.6792$).

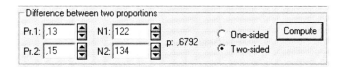

Since 0.6792 is higher than the critical significance level of 0.05, we accept the null hypothesis. Thus, there is no statistically significant differences in lethality under halothane and morphine anesthesia ($p = 0.6792$).

The construction of the confidence interval for the difference of the relative frequencies in the case of independent samples is considered in 2.3 and p.8.1.5. To find the quantile t you can use *Probability calculator*.

Note. *In case when the studied feature is observed as 0% or 100% in one of the groups, it is necessary to input not 0 or 1 but the numbers which are close to them, for example, 0.00000000001 or 0.9999999 to calculate the significance test in the software package Statistica. This change does not affect the results of the calculations.*

CHAPTER 6

THE APPLICATION OF THE STATISTICA SOFTWARE PACKAGE FOR DEPENDENCES ANALYSIS

6.1. DEPENDENCE ANALYSIS (CORRELATIONS, ASSOCIATIONS)

PARAMETRIC AND NON-PARAMETRIC CORRELATIONS

The choice of correlation coefficient directly depends on the measurement scale within which variables, numbers of changeable characteristics in compared variables and variables distributions are measured. Consider the table of criteria to detect the dependences between variables expressed in different scales. In this research we turn the attention only on those which are widely used in the analysis of medical information.

Table 6-1

The criteria to carry out correlation analysis

Scale type		Criterion
Variable X	Variable Y	
Interval or ratio scale	Interval or ratio scale	Pearson's coefficient (normal distribution)
Ordinal, interval or ratio scale	Ordinal, interval or ratio scale	Spearman's coefficient (abnormal distribution)
Ordinal	Ordinal	τ-Kendall gamma criterion
Dichotomous	Dichotomous	φ coefficient; χ^2 Yates corrected Chi-square Fisher's exact test
Dichotomous	Ordinal	r_{rb} rank-biserial coefficient
Dichotomous	Interval or ratio scale	r_{bis} biserial coefficient
Interval or ratio scale	Dichotomous	r_{pb} point biserial coefficient

If one of the two related variables has ratio or interval scale and is normally distributed, Pearson's parametric criterion is used. If at least one of the two related variables has ordinal scale or abnormal distribution (at a ratio or interval scale), Spearman's rank correlation, Kendall rank correlation coefficient (τ-Kendall) or χ^2 and Fisher's criteria which have been considered in **5.2** are used instead of Pearson's criterion.

Spearman rank correlation coefficient (r-Spearman) is a non-parametric analogue of the classical Pearson correlation coefficient between ranks without taking into account arithmetical average and variance. It is computed with the following formula:

$$r_s = 1 - \frac{6 \cdot \sum d^2}{n^3 - n},$$

where d is the difference between ranks for each member of the sample.

Testing statistical hypothesis, order of statistical decision making and formulating valuable conclusions are the same as for r –Pearson. The levels of statistical significance for the same coefficients r –Pearson and r-Spearman always coincide in computer programs. If parametric

113

methods requiring normal distribution are applied to the data of a different distribution type, it will lead to the false conclusion. On the contrary, non-parametric methods can be used in case of normal distribution. However, their sensitivity will be much lower. In terms of Spearman's rank correlation coefficient, it is left slightly behind Pearson's r coefficient. The advantage of r-Spearman over r –Pearson consists in higher sensitivity in the following cases:

• in significant distribution violations of at least one variable from a standard form (asymmetry, outlying cases);

• in case of curvilinear (monotonic) relationship

The application of r-Spearman coefficient is restricted by

• the number of observations of every variable which is less than 5;

• a great number of equal ranks, when a coefficient gives rough value.

Kendall's τ- coefficient

Sir Maurice Kendall, a British statistician, suggested a simple method to calculate the correlation. Suppose that there are the data of the same objects evaluated by two users. In order to determine the correlation coefficient between these objects we will find the difference be-tween x_1-x_2 and y_1-y_2 for all paired estimates (x_1, x_2) и (y_1, y_2), where x is the estimates of one user, and y is the estimates of another one. A pair of two variables is considered to be *concordant* when two differences have equal signs. If the signs are different, the pair is regarded as *discon-cordant*. The correlation is characterized by the value $S = P - Q$ where P is the number of con-cordant pairs, while Q is the number of disconcordant ones (inversions). The larger S is, the more alike the compared objects are. We divide S by a number of possible pairs $n(n-1)/2$, where n is the number of examined objects, for the results to be easily analyzed. We obtain the following formula:

$$\tau = \frac{2S}{n(n-1)} = \frac{2P}{n(n-1)} - \frac{2Q}{n(n-1)}$$

The parameter normalized in such a way will be changed in the range $-1 < \tau < 1$. If $\tau=1$, then the objects are the same; if $\tau =-1$, they are opposite; if $\tau = 0$, they have nothing in common. Kendall's tau (τ) can also be interpreted in terms of probability. The first summand is the prob-ability that pairs are concordant (objects are alike). The second summand is the probability of pair disconcordance. Hence, we examine whether there is a difference between probabilities. The sum of these summands results in total probabilities equal to 1. Kendall's tau (τ) is equivalent to r-Spearman if some basic assumptions are fulfilled. Their powers are also equivalent. It is widely accepted that τ-Kendall provides the complete and detailed analysis of the relations between va-riables sorting out all possible correspondences between pairs of values.

There are two types of the τ-Kendall statistics: *tau-b* and *tau-c*. They differ in the way of handling tied ranks. In most cases their values are quite similar. If there are differences, the lower of the two values is considered.

Gamma criterion

Gamma statistics is more preferable than r-Spearman or τ-Kendall if the data have many common values. In terms of basic assumptions, Gamma statistics, its interpretation and calcula-tions are more similar to the τ-Kendall than to the r-Spearman statistics except the coincidences which are taken into account in normalizing. Gamma represents the difference between the prob-ability that the rank order of two variables coincides and the probability that it does not coincide divided by one minus coincidence probability.

Coefficient φ

While comparing two variables measured on a dichotomous scale, **φ coefficient** serves as a correlation measure. Dichotomous data are arranged in a four-field contingency table.

			Variable X	
			0	1
Variable Y		1	a	b
		0	c	d

The coefficient is calculated by the following formula:

$$\varphi = \frac{bc - ad}{\sqrt{(a+c)(b+d)(a+b)(c+d)}}$$

where a is the number of items with code 0 for x and 1 for y; b is the number of items with code 1 for x and 1 for y; c is the number of items with code 0 for x and 0 for y; d is the number of items with code 1 for x and 0 for y.

The number of all items in the sample $n=a+b+c+d$.

The values of the coefficient φ range from +1 to -1. Its values characterize not only the strength of the relations, but also the direction of the relation between two dichotomously measured variables. However, the interpretation of φ may cause specific problems.

If the variable x is measured on a dichotomous scale, but y is measured on an ordinal scale, the rank-biserial correlation coefficient may be used

$$r_{rb} = \frac{\bar{y}_1 - \bar{y}_0}{n/2}\ ,$$

where $\bar{y}_1$ – the y average rank which corresponds to the code 1 in the variable x; $\bar{y}_0$ – the y average rank which corresponds to the code 0 in the variable x; n – the number of all items in the sample.

This coefficient is closely connected with τ-Kendall and uses the concepts of concordance and inversion in its definition.

Biserial correlation coefficient

The biserial correlation coefficient is used when one variable, for instance x, is measured on a dichotomous scale, while the other variable, y as an example, is measured on an interval or ratio scale. Testing the hypothesis about the influence of a child's gender on height and weight, indicators may serve as an example. The variable y must have normal distribution law.

The biserial correlation coefficient:

$$r_{bis} = \frac{\bar{y}_1 - \bar{y}_0}{S_y}\sqrt{\frac{n_1 n_0}{n(n-1)}}\ ,$$

where n_0 is the number of items with the score of 0, n_1 is the number of the items with the score of 1; $\bar{y}_1$ is the average over those elements of the variable y, which corresponds to the code 1 in the variable x; $\bar{y}_0$ is the average on those elements of the variable y, which corresponds to the code 0 in the variable x; S_y is the standard deviation of y.

The coefficient ranges from -1 to +1, but its sign makes no difference for the results interpretation.

The point biserial correlation coefficient is used when one variable (y as an example) is dichotomous and the other variable x is measured on an interval or ratio scale. The variable x must be normally distributed.

The point biserial correlation coefficient is:

$$r_{pb} = \frac{\bar{x}_1 - \bar{x}_0}{S_x} \sqrt{\frac{n_1 n_0}{n(n-1)}}$$

where n_0 is the number of items with the score of 0, n_1 is the number of the items with the score of 1; $\bar{x}_1$ is the average over those elements of the variable x, which corresponds to the code 1 in the variable y; $\bar{x}_0$ is the average over those elements of the variable x, which corresponds to the code 0 in the variable y; S_x is the standard deviation of x.

The coefficient ranges from -1 to +1, but its sign makes no difference for the results interpretation.

*Note. All coefficients are significantly tested using the same formula of the criterion as Pearson's coefficient. The critical point of Student's quantile is found either from the Student's table or by **the Probability calculator** in the Statistica package.*

Consider the specific examples of different correlation cases.

6.1.1. THE PEARSON CORRELATION COEFFICIENT

Example 6.1. The relation between age and arterial blood pressure

There are the data about age and arterial blood pressure of some patients. Do the obtained data indicate the relations between them? Let us state the statistic hypotheses.

Null hypothesis H_0: there are no relations between the variables.

Table 6-2

Age and Arterial Blood Pressure

	1 age	2 blood pressure
Ivanov	40	145
Petrov	48	127
Sidorov	30	130
Kozlov	25	120
Karpov	41	140
Skvorzov	43	135
Kovalev	50	145
Sotnikov	60	150
Rethkov	55	140
Popov	34	130
Sokolov	65	155
Smekov	30	125

Work order

1. Launch the program *Statistica*.

2. Enter the data as they are arranged in the table. Denote the variables as **age** and **blood pressure.** Test the variable normal distribution with the help of **Descriptive Statistics** to justify the use of r –Pearson.

3. Click on *Statistics – Basic Statistic and Tables* after the results about normal distribution are obtained. Choose *Correlation matrices.* Click *OK.*

4. Click the tab *Options* and select *Display r-level and N's.* Click on **OK/Summary.**

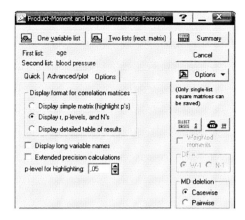

5. Enter the variables. *The first variable list –*age, *the second variable list (optional) –* *blood pressure*. Click *OK*.

The analysis table which indicates the correlation coefficient 0.8357 and the level of significance which is less than critical (0.001) will appear. The results show that the correlation is strong and direct. In other words, blood pressure increases with age.

Variable	Correlations (Pearson) Marked correlations are significant at p < ,05000 N=12 (Casewise deletion of missing data) blood pressure
age	,8357
	p= ,001

6. Close down the analysis table. Click the tab *Advanced/Plot* and the button **2D Scatterplots.** The scatterplot will be displayed which visually demonstrates that the relation between the parameters is strong as the cloud is drawn along the trend line. Two values are beyond 95% of the confidence interval. Close the window.

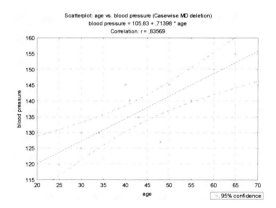

6.1.2. THE SPEARMAN CORRELATION COEFFICIENT

Example 6.2.[6].

Chlorhexidine oral rinse prevents from plague and has taste far from being pleasant. Besides, it is teeth dying. Sal ammoniac mouthwash has a nice taste and is not teeth dying, but less

117

effective. F.P. Ashley and collaborators compared these two kinds of mouthwash. They estimated dental plague visually in points and by weighing after removal. The results are presented in the table.

Table 6-3

The amount of dental plague estimated visually in points and by weighing

Visual estimate in points	Weight of dry dental plague in mg
25	2.7
32	1.2
45	2.7
60	2.1
60	3.5
65	2.8
68	3.7
78	8.9
80	5.8
83	4
100	5.1
110	5.1
120	4.8
125	5.8
140	11.7
143	8.5
143	11.1
145	7.4
148	14.2
153	12.2

Is the visual method of estimation reliable, judging from these data? We suggest a null hypothesis H_0 about the absence of the relations between the visual estimates and the results of weighing as well as the alternative hypothesis H_1 which states that the relations between the variables exist.

Work order

1. Launch the program *Statistica.*

2. Enter the data as they are arranged in the table. Denote the variables as *points* and *weight*. The Spearman criterion should be used as one variable is ordinal.

3. Click *Statistics – Nonparametrics* in the options menu. Choose *Correlations (Spearman, Kendall tau, gamma).* Click *OK.*

4. In the field *Compute* of the appeared window choose *Detailed report*, click *Variables* and enter the variables. *The first variable list is points, the second variable list is weight.* Click *Spearman rank R.*

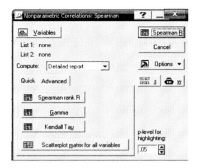

The analysis table will be displayed which indicates the correlation coefficient 0.8888 and the level of significance 0.0000. The results show that the correlation is strong and direct. Hence, the visual estimate corresponds to the weighing results quite well.

	Spearman Rank Order Correlations (Spearman) MD pairwise deleted Marked correlations are significant at p <,05000			
Pair of Variables	Valid N	Spearman R	t(N-2)	p-level
points & weight	20	0,888889	8,231935	0,000000

Example 6.3.[6]. The correlation between the level of sickle-cell disease serenity and the coefficient of red blood cells adhesion.

Sickle-cell disease leads to red cells deformation, blood vessel embolism and hypoxia. There is an assumption that it is caused not only by erythrocyte deformation, but also by predisposition to adhesion - to endothelium. To estimate the level of serenity, different signs of the disease were summarized. The level of serenity and the adhesion coefficient were estimated for 20 examined patients. Points for particular signs of the disease were summarized in the way that every patient got from 0 to 13 points or more (2 points are given for every heart attack or avascular necrosis).

To estimate the adhesion, the cultured endothelium was covered with the known quantity of erythrocytes, and then erythrocytes were incubated and washed away. Having counted the quantity of washed erythrocytes, the number of adhered erythrocytes was defined. The same experiment was carried out with normal erythrocyte level. The results were expressed by the coefficient of adhesion: the ratio between the numbers of adhered erythrocytes of a sick and of a healthy person.

Do these data prove the hypothesis about the correlation between erythrocyte adhesion and the level of sickle-cell disease serenity?

We suggest a null hypothesis H_0 about the absence of relations between adhesion and the level of serenity as well as an alternative hypothesis H_1 about the correlation between the variables with the level of significance 0.05. The Spearman coefficient is used in the analysis as one variable is ordinal.

Table 6-4

The level of sickle-cell disease serenity
and the coefficient of erythrocyte adhesion

The level of the disease serenity (in points)	The factor of adhesion
0	1.0
0	1.4
1	1.0
1	1.0
1	1.9
1	2.0
1	2.5
1	3.0
2	2.0
2	3.2
3	3.0
3	3.2
3	6.3
4	2.7
5	3.0
5	5.0
5	17.0
6	5.2
9	19.8
11	25.0

Work order

1. Launch the program *Statistica*.

2. Enter the data. Denote the variables as *points* and *factor*. Click *Statistics – Nonparametrics* in the options menu. Select *Correlations (Spearman, Kendall tau, gamma)*. Click *OK*.

3. In the field *Compute* of the appeared window *Nonparametric Correlations* choose *Detailed report*, click *Variables* and enter the data. *The first variable list is points, the second variable list is factor.* Click *Spearman rank R*. The analysis table will be displayed.

	Spearman Rank Order Correlations (Spearman_2) MD pairwise deleted Marked correlations are significant at p <,05000			
Pair of Variables	Valid N	Spearman R	t(N-2)	p-level
points & factor	20	0,861114	7,185906	0,000001

The analysis table shows that Spearman's rank correlation coefficient equals 0.86 and the level of significance is 0.000001. The data prove the alternative hypothesis about the correlations between the erythrocyte adhesion and the level of the disease serenity.

Note. *Having several predictors to check whether they correlate with each other or not, the same independent variables are to be chosen after clicking Variables.*

This example can be solved by the τ-Kendall criterion.

Close the table, return to the window *Nonparametric Correlations*, click the tab *Advanced*. Click on *Kendall Tau*. The table confirming the alternative hypothesis about the correlations between the erythrocyte adhesion and the level of the disease serenity will be displayed. Close the window.

Pair of Variables	Kendall Tau Correlations (Spearman_2) MD pairwise deleted Marked correlations are significant at p <,05000				
	Valid **N**	Kendall Tau	Z	p-level	p-exact 1-tailed
points & factor	20	0,734203	4,525930	0,000006	----

6.1.3. KENDALL'S COEFFICIENT OF CONCORDANCE

Spearman's coefficient as well as τ-Kendall can be applied to find out the experts' consistency of opinions. But there is one more kind of rank correlation coefficient which is called as **Kendall's coefficient of concordance W** (Kendall's concordance W). In contrast to the Spearman rank coefficient, it can be extended to a number of independent variables to measure the degree of consistency between multiple related samples. Kendall's concordance W was introduced to carry out tests in the situation when a large number of respondents expresses their opinions concerning a great number of observed persons (objects). In this case observed objects form separate variables, while observers – individual observations which will be compared with each other. The coefficient of concordance W indicates the degree of unanimity among the respondents. For instance, a psychologist studying the attitude towards family life asks to range some personal qualities which are crucial for the well-being of the family. W- Kendall's is more preferable, if there are outlying cases in the initial data. The concordance coefficient ranges from 0 to 1 (0 < W < 1), where 0 means no agreement and 1 is complete agreement. Its formula is as follows:

$$W = \frac{12S}{n(m^3 - m)},$$

where S is the sum of the squares of the deviations of total rank estimates of every object under examination from the average value; n – number of experts and m – number of objects.

Example 6.4. .[4]. The concordance of experts' opinions

Suppose that seven experts estimated the level publications in five medical journals giving them from 1 to 6 points. Is it possible to evaluate significant differences between the magazines based on the experts' estimates? Are these experts reliable? Suggest a null hypothesis H_0 about the absence of differences and an alternative hypothesis H_1 about the existence of differences, namely, about the correlation between the level of publications and the magazine with the level of significance 0.05.

	1 m_1	2 m_2	3 m_3	4 m_4	5 m_5
Smirnov	1	2	3	4	6
Ivanov	6	1	4	3	2
Petrov	3	2	1	6	4
Kirillov	3	2	6	1	4
Avanesov	2	1	6	4	3
Matrosov	1	3	6	2	4
Schubin	2	3	1	6	4

Work order

1. Launch the program *Statistica.* Denote the variables *m_1, ... m_5* and enter their values.

2. Click *Statistics – Nonparametrics* in the options menu. Choose *Comparing multiple dependant samples (variables).* Click *OK.*

3. In the appeared window click *Variables* and choose the variables from *m_1* to *m_5.* Click on *OK.*

4. Click on *Summary: Friedman ANOVA & Kendall's concordance* in the window *Friedman ANOVA by Ranks.* As the estimates in points are ordinal, χ^2 can be used to reveal the differences between the magazines, while the level of experts' concordance is checked by *Kendall's concordance W.*

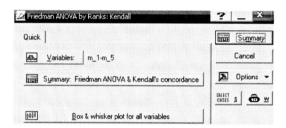

The table with the data analysis will appear.

Variable	Friedman ANOVA and Kendall Coeff. of Concordance (Kendal ANOVA Chi Sqr. (N = 7, df = 4) = 6,171429 p = ,18671 Coeff. of Concordance = ,22041 Aver. rank r = ,09048			
	Average Rank	Sum of Ranks	Mean	Std.Dev.
m_1	2,428571	17,00000	2,571429	1,718249
m_2	2,000000	14,00000	2,000000	0,816497
m_3	3,428571	24,00000	3,857143	2,267787
m_4	3,428571	24,00000	3,714286	1,889822
m_5	3,714286	26,00000	3,857143	1,214986

The table shows that the alternative hypothesis is rejected; the null hypothesis is accepted. In experts' opinion there are no significant differences between the magazines, as χ^2 is equal to 6.17 with the level of significance $p < 0.18671$. However, the sum of ranks shows that *m_1* and *m_2* differ from *m_3, m_4, m_5.* The second magazine has the least sum of ranks. The level of experts' concordance of opinions is low as the concordance of coefficient is 0.22.

Conclusion: the quality of publications does not depend on the magazine. Close the window.

5. Click on the *Box & whisker plot for all variables* button, choose *Median/Quart./Range* for graphs, then click *Ok.*

The diagram denotes the differences between the first and second magazines as well as the third, fourth and fifth ones.

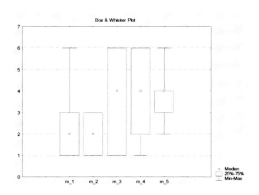

Box & Whisker Plot

6.2. THE METHODS OF REGRESSION ANALYSIS

6.2.1. MULTIPLE LINEAR REGRESSION

Example 6.5. The relations between anthropometric data
Compare the tables of patients' information concerning weight, age, systolic pressure and diastolic pressure.
Work order
1. Launch the program *Statistica*.

	1 pressure/sys	2 pressure/dias	3 weight	4 age
Ivanov	145	72	75	40
Petrova	127	65	70	48
Smirnova	130	70	65	30
Koylov	120	65	75	25
Orlov	140	80	85	41
Fedorova	135	90	60	43
Stepanova	145	85	70	50
Belov	150	80	78	60
Blinov	140	75	85	55
Adamov	130	77	60	34
Ozerov	155	80	72	65
Pavlov	125	68	80	30

2. Enter the data, denote the variables.

3. Click *Statistics – Basic Statistics/Tables* in the options menu. Choose *Correlation matrices*. Click *OK*.

4. In a new window click *One variable list*. In the opened window enter all four variables. Click *OK*.

5. Choose the tab *Options* and set up a switch on *Display r, p-levels and N's*.

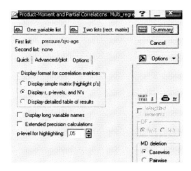

6. Click on *Summary* to view correlation coefficient matrix.

123

Variable	Correlations (Multi_regression) Marked correlations are significant at p < ,05000 N=12 (Casewise deletion of missing data)			
	pressure/sys	pressure/dias	weight	age
pressure/sys	1,0000	,6135	,1951	,8357
	p= ---	p=,034	p=,543	p=,001
pressure/dias	,6135	1,0000	-,2387	,4847
	p=,034	p= ---	p=,455	p=,110
weight	,1951	-,2387	1,0000	,2004
	p=,543	p=,455	p= ---	p=,532
age	,8357	,4847	,2004	1,0000
	p=,001	p=,110	p=,532	p= ---

The most significant correlation coefficients ($p<0.05$) are highlighted in red in the matrix. The correlation between the variables pressure/sys and age is the strongest in this case. The coefficient is equal to 0.8357 with the significance point 0.001. The weight of a patient correlates with no indicators. Also, pressure/sys correlates with pressure/dias. The correlation coefficient equals 0.6135 with the level of significance 0.034. Close the window.

7. Click on the *Advanced/Plot* tab and press the *Scatterplot Matrix* button, display the graphic data. Choose the same variables.

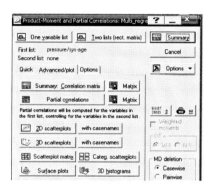

The matrix indicates that the largest angle of inclination, which points to the greatest correlation coefficient in the diagram, is lying at the intersection of the line *age* and the column *systolic pressure*.

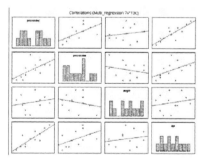

Close the window. Having analyzed the correlations between the variables, pass on to multiple regression model making. Start from the case when there is only one independent variable (predictor). It will be *pressure/dias*. *Pressure/sys* will be a dependant variable. Further, we will introduce other predictors *(age and weight)* to improve the model.

Regression model for two variables (systolic and diastolic pressure)

1. Close all windows except the window with initial data used to make a correlation matrix. Choose *Statistics – Multiple Regression* in the options menu.

2. Press *Variables* in the *Multiple Linear Regression* window, click on the tab *Advanced* and denote *Dependent variable* as *pressure/sys*, *Independent variable* as *pressure/dias*. Click *Ok*. The window allowing choosing variables will be closed.

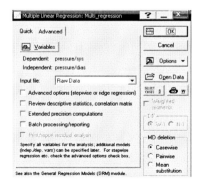

3. Pressing on *Ok* in the *Multiple Linear Regression* window will call up the *Multiple Regression Results* window.

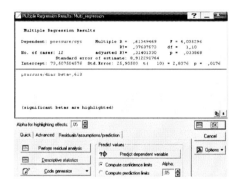

The title from the top of the window indicates that the quality of this model is not high as the determination coefficient R^2=0.376. However, the model is valid with the significant point p<0.034.

4. Choose the tab *Quick* and press on the *Summary: Regression results* to display the following table:

	Regression Summary for Dependent Variable: pressure/sys (Mu R= ,61349469 R?= ,37637573 Adjusted R?= ,31401330 F(1,10)=6,0353 p<,03387 Std.Error of estimate: 8,9123					
N=12	**Beta**	Std.Err. of Beta	B	Std.Err. of B	t(10)	p-level
Intercept			73,50750	25,90503	2,837577	0,017621
pressure/dias	0,613495	0,249725	0,83783	0,34104	2,456684	0,033868

Determination coefficient and the level of significance are indicated in the title of the table. The second line of the table contains the information which allows predicting the dependent variable through the independent one using linear regression equation $y=bx+a_0$, as the model is linear. In this case the absolute term of the equation is a_0=73.5. The angular coefficient is b=0.837. Then, *pressure /sys* =73.5075+0.83783×*pressure/dias*. For instance, for *pressure/dias*. **(Ivanov)**=72 the predicted value *pressure/sys* =73.5075+0.83783×72=133.83 is obtained. Similar prediction can be done with the help of the *Predict dependent variable* button. Close the table.

5. Choose the tab *Residuals/assumptions/prediction* in the window *Multiple Regression Results*. Click on *Predict dependent variable.*

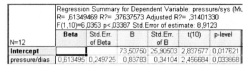

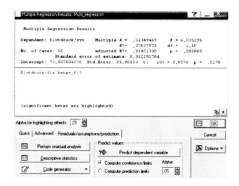

6. Enter the *pressure/dias* value in the window which is equal to 72 and click *Ok*.

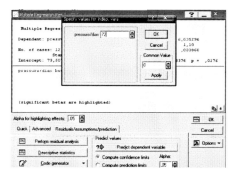

The following table will be displayed:

Variable	Predicting Values for (Multi_regre variable: pressure/sys		
	B-Weight	Value	B-Weight * Value
pressure/dias	0,837828	72,00000	60,3236
Intercept			73,5075
Predicted			133,8311
-95,0%CL			127,4848
+95,0%CL			140,1774

The predicted *pressure/sys* makes 133.83. The limits of confidence interval constitute 127.48 – 140.17 with confidence coefficient of 95%. Besides, weight coefficients to calculate predicted values are given in the first lines of the last column (73.507+60.323=133.83).

The determination coefficient is low. It means that pressure/sys can be influenced by other predictors. Let us improve the regression model by introducing the predictors *age* and *weight*.

Regression model with a set of predictors

1. Return to the window with initial data and close other windows. Choose *Statistics – Multiple Regression* in the options menu to open the *Multiple Linear Regression* window.

2. Press the tab *Advanced* and the button *Variables* in the appeared window, denote *Dependent var.(or list for batch) – pressure/sys, Independent variable list – pressure/dias., weigt, age.* Click *OK*.

126

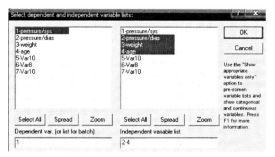

3. Press on Ok in the window ***Multiple Linear Regression*** to get the results of the analysis:

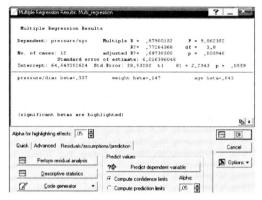

The top of the window indicates that the model is improved, but describes our data unsatisfactory: R^2=0.7726 p<0.005946.

4. Choose the tab ***Residuals/assumptions/prediction*** and press on ***Descriptive statistics***. In the appeared window choose the tab ***Quick*** and click on ***Correlations***.

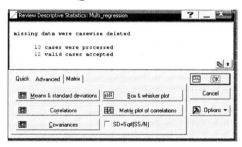

The following table will appear:

Variable	Correlations (Multi_regression)			
	pressure/dias	weight	age	pressure/sys
pressure/dias	1,000000	-0,238683	0,484678	0,613495
weight	-0,238683	1,000000	0,200394	0,195116
age	0,484678	0,200394	1,000000	0,835689
pressure/sys	0,613495	0,195116	0,835689	1,000000

The table shows that the predictors are not connected with each other (the correlation coefficients are less than 0.5). However, ***pressure/sys*** except ***pressure/dias*** is influenced by **age** (the coefficients 0.61 and 0.83). This result was obtained in the correlation matrix. Close the window.

5. Return to the ***Multiple Regression Results*** window, choose the tab ***Advanced*** and click on ***Summary: Regression results***. The analysis table will be displayed on the screen.

N=12	Regression Summary for Dependent Variable: pressure/sys (Mu R= ,87900152 R?= ,77264368 Adjusted R?= ,68738505 F(3,8)=9,0624 p<,00595 Std.Error of estimate: 6,0164					
	Beta	Std.Err. of Beta	B	Std.Err. of B	t(8)	p-level
Intercept			64,64335	28,93202	2,234319	0,055919
pressure/dias	0,336825	0,209486	0,45999	0,28609	1,607865	0,146532
weight	0,146647	0,187030	0,18610	0,23734	0,784086	0,455576
age	0,643050	0,207643	0,54940	0,17740	3,096903	0,014735

The model looks in the following way.

The absolute term of the equation is equal to 64.64335 in the *B* column. The coefficients of those variables which are predictors or independent variables are arranged in lines below the value of the absolute term of the equation in the *B* column. The regression equation allows calculating *pressure/sys* based on the known values of the *age, pressure/dias* and *weight* variables. The pressure/sys value for the first patient will be:

pressure/sys = 64.64335+0.45999×(*pressure/dias*)+0.1861×(*weight.*)+0.5494×(*age*)=133.696.

The last regression table indicates that the levels of significance of some variables included in the table exceed 0.05. It means that not all variables should be included in the table. Close the windows.

6. Choose the *Residuals/assumptions/prediction* tab in the *Multiple Regression Results* window. Click *Ok* to view the *Residual Analysis* table:

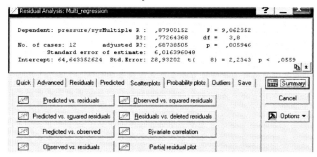

7. Press *Advanced* and *Summary: Residuals & predicted.* There will be the values of the variable and its predicted values arranged in the table.

Case No.	Observed Value	Predicted Value	Residual	Standard Pred. v.	Standard Residual	Std.Err. Pred.Val	Mahalanobis Distance	Deleted Residual	Cook's Distance
Ivanov	145,0000	133,6956	11,30437	-0,33173	1,87893	1,951776	0,240990	12,6340	0,116021
Petrova	127,0000	133,9404	-6,94040	-0,30586	-1,15358	4,259278	4,596382	-13,9138	0,670129
Smirnova	130,0000	125,4207	4,57926	-1,20660	0,76113	3,087296	1,979852	6,2161	0,070272
Koylov	120,0000	122,2348	-2,23476	-1,54344	-0,37145	3,472460	2,747661	-3,3511	0,025837
Orlov	140,0000	139,7859	0,21410	0,31216	0,03559	4,169283	4,365870	0,4119	0,000563
Fedorova	135,0000	140,8322	-5,83220	0,42278	-0,96938	4,437801	5,068214	-12,7922	0,614919
Stepanova	145,0000	144,2390	0,76102	0,78296	0,12649	2,781232	1,434017	0,9678	0,001383
Belov	150,0000	148,9218	1,07825	1,27805	0,17922	3,019185	1,853458	1,4412	0,003613
Blinov	140,0000	145,1775	-5,17751	0,88219	-0,86057	3,333839	2,460940	-7,4717	0,118393
Adamov	130,0000	129,9078	0,09222	-0,73221	0,01533	3,367838	2,530182	0,1343	0,000039
Ozerov	155,0000	150,5522	4,44783	1,45043	0,73928	3,782812	3,431932	7,3558	0,147734
Pavlov	125,0000	127,2922	-2,29219	-1,00874	-0,38099	3,248635	2,290501	-3,2355	0,021081
Minimum	120,0000	122,2348	-6,94040	-1,54344	-1,15358	1,951776	0,240990	-13,9138	0,000039
Maximum	155,0000	150,5522	11,30437	1,45043	1,87893	4,437801	5,068214	12,6340	0,670129
Mean	136,8333	136,8333	-0,00000	0,00000	-0,00000	3,409286	2,750000	-0,9669	0,149165
Median	137,5000	136,8632	0,15316	0,00315	0,02546	3,350839	2,495561	0,2731	0,048054

For instance, the measured value of *pressure/sys* for the first patient is 145, but the predicted value is 133.6956. Close the table and the *Residual Analysis* window. Close down the window.

8. Press *Ok* in the *Multiple Linear Regression* window. Click on the *Residuals/assumptions/ prediction* tab and the *Predict dependent variable* button in the *Multiple Re-*

gression Results window. Enter the data of the first patient in the appeared window: *pressure/dias* -72, *age* – 75, *weight* – 40. Click *OK*.

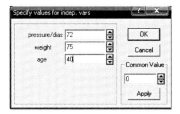

The predicted value of systolic pressure equal to 133.6956 will be shown in the next table. The confidence interval of predicted values (the lowest limit is 129.1948, the highest limit is 138.1964) is indicated as well. Besides, the first lines of the last column show weight coefficients to calculate the predicted value (33.1193+13.9572+21.9758+64.6434=133.6956).

Variable	Predicting Values for (Multi_regression) variable: pressure/sys		
	B-Weight	Value	B-Weight * Value
pressure/dias	0,459990	72,00000	33,1193
weight	0,186096	75,00000	13,9572
age	0,549396	40,00000	21,9758
Intercept			64,6434
Predicted			133,6956
-95,0%CL			129,1948
+95,0%CL			138,1964

As the model does not predict the values of the variables exactly, and the determination coefficient is not high R^2=0.7726, let us still improve the model applying step-by-step method. It consists in including or excluding an independent variable at every step of the model. Hence, multiple valuable significant variables are singled out. It allows reducing the number of variables which describe the dependence. The variables which are not valuable for the model are excluded.

Work order

1. Close all windows and return to the initial data. Choose *Statistics – Multiple Regression* in the options menu. Press on *Variables*. Choose the dependent variable *pressure/sys* in the left window and independent predictors *pressure/dias, weight* **and** *age* in the right window. Set the option *Advanced options (stepwise or ridge regression)*. Click *Ok*.

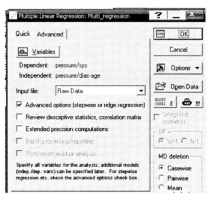

2. Choose *Advanced* in the *Model Definition* window and *Forward stepwise* in the field *Method* for better variable selection. Press *Ok*.

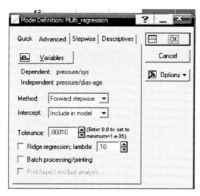

The **Multiple Regression Results** window will show that the variable age is more significant as it is red, and the level of significance for the model does not exceed 0.05. However, the determination coefficient is low (R^2 = 0.755).

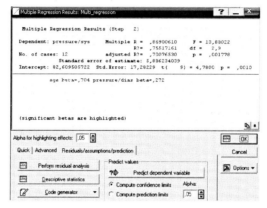

3. Choose the tab **Advanced** and click **Summary: Regression Results** to view the coefficient matrix.

N=12	Beta	Std.Err. of Beta	B	Std.Err. of B	t(9)	p-level
Intercept			82,60951	17,28229	4,780008	0,001001
age	0,703634	0,188562	0,60116	0,16110	3,731582	0,004686
pressure/dias	0,272459	0,188562	0,37209	0,25751	1,444931	0,182378

Regression Summary for Dependent Variable: pressure/sys (M
R= ,86900610 R?= ,75517161 Adjusted R?= ,70076530
F(2,9)=13,880 p<,00178 Std.Error of estimate: 5,8862

The table indicates that only **age** and **pressure/dias** are taken into account (non-significant variable **weight** is excluded). Consider the level of significance which is lower than 0.05 for **age** and higher than 0.05 for the predictor **pressure/dias**. It specifies its small contribution to the model. The program calculated a new value of the absolute term of the equation which equals 82.60951, the linear equation coefficients of the predictors **age** and **pressure/dias** which make 0.60116 and 0.37209, respectively. In this case, the regression equation looks as follows:

pressure/sys = 82.60951+0.60116×**age** +0.37209×**pressure/dias**

Let us substitute the value into the equation to predict the first case:

pressure/sys = 82.60951+0.60116×40+0.37209×72 = 133.44.

Close the table.

4. Return to **Multiple Regression Results**, click the tab **Residuals/assumptions/prediction** and press on the **Perform residual analysis** button to display the **Residual analysis** window.

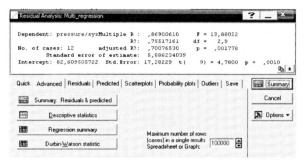

5. Click on the tab *Probability plots*. Press the *Normal plot of residuals* button to make a graph.

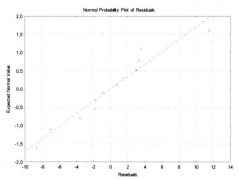

As it has been already mentioned above, multiple regression suggests that there are linear inter-variable relation in equation and normal distribution of residuals. If these assumptions are violated, the conclusion can be inexact. The normal probability plot of residuals will point out whether there are any serious violations of these assumptions or not.

This plot is produced in the following way. At first, standard residuals are ranged in order. The z or t values (meaning the standard normal distribution values) can be calculated using these ranks based on the assumption that the data are subjected to the normal distribution. The z or t values are plotted on the y-axis. If the observed residuals (plotted along the x-axis) are normally distributed, all values will lay off as a straight line on the plot. All points of our plot lay close to the line. If the residuals are not normally distributed, they diverge from a straight line. Also outlying cases become noticeable on the graph. The graph shows that measurements with residuals of 3 and 11.5 are outlying cases which can distort the analysis. Close the window.

6. Choose the tab *Residuals* in the *Residual Analysis* window and press on the *Histogram of residuals* button.

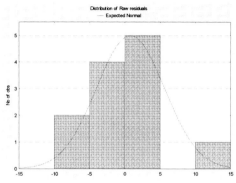

The histogram of residuals distribution can be indicative of the model adequacy. Adequate model is characterized by the residual distribution close to the normal law. Unfortunately, the Statistica package does not allow using statistical tests in this module, but the graph denotes that there are some non-significant violations of the normal distribution. Close the window.

As the determination coefficient of the model R^2=0.755 is not high, it points to the poor quality of the model. At this point a linear regression model is used up.

6.2.2. MULTIPLE NONLINEAR REGRESSION

Multiple nonlinear regression is applied when simple linear regression model inadequately reflects variables dependence.

Work order

1. Close all the windows to change the model and return to the initial data. Select *Statistics – Advanced Linear/Nonlinear Models – Fixed Nonlinear Regression* in the options menu.

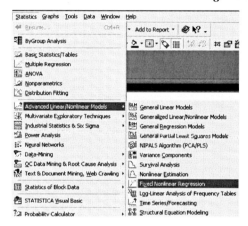

2. Click on *Variables* in the appeared *Fixed Nonlinear Regression* window. Denote the examined variables (not more than four). Press *Ok*. Click on *Ok* one more time.

3. Select the options for nonlinear functions X**2 and X**3 (X to the second power; X to the third power) in the appeared *Nonlinear Components Regression* window. Click *Ok*.

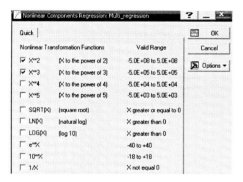

4. Select *Variables* in a new window. Denote the first variable named 1- *pressure/sys* in the *Dependent variables* field. Mark all variables except **1-*pressure/sys*, 5-*V1***2, 6-*V1***3** (except the dependent variable, its square and cube). Perform the operations holding down *Ctrl*. Click *Ok*.

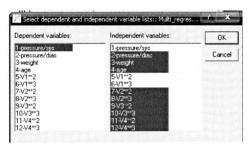

5. Choose the *Advanced* tab in the *Model Definition* window and *Forward stepwise* in the *Method* field. Press on *Ok*.

The *Multiple Regression Results* window will be displayed. The window indicates that the determination coefficient of this model makes 0.8588 with the significant point 0.000919. It means that the observed results are well-described by the model.

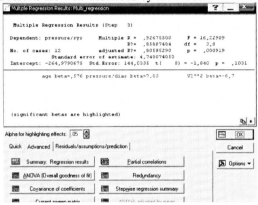

6. Press on the *Advanced* tab and the *Summary: Regression results* button to display the table to make an equation.

N=12	Regression Summary for Dependent Variable: pressure/sys (Mu R= ,92675500 R?= ,85887484 Adjusted R?= ,80595290 F(3,8)=16,229 p<,00092 Std.Error of estimate: 4,7401					
	Beta	Std.Err. of Beta	B	Std.Err. of B	t(8)	p-level
Intercept			-264,979	144,0335	-1,83970	0,103092
age	0,57604	0,160706	0,492	0,1373	3,58442	0,007142
pressure/dias	7,03475	2,793171	9,607	3,8145	2,51855	0,035890
V2**2	-6,70911	2,767107	-0,060	0,0247	-2,42459	0,041551

After the step-by-step analysis those variables which contribute the most into the model are left in the first column. These variables are *age, pressure/dias* and *V2**2* (it is *pressure/dias* squared). The *B* column contains the information for making an equation. The absolute term of the equation is equal to 264.979; the *age* variable coefficient makes 0.492; the *pressure/dias* variable coefficient is 9.607; the coefficient of the *pressure/dias squared* (*V2**2*) variable equals -0.060. Hence, the equation looks as follows:

pressure/sys = -264.979 + 0.492× *age* + 9.607×*pressure/dias.* $-.060 \times (pressure/dias.)^2$.

7. Close the table. Select the *Residuals/assumptions/prediction* tab and press the *Perform residual analysis* button to observe the *Residual Analysis* window.

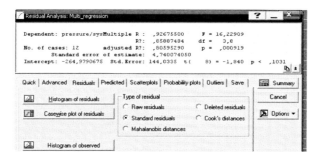

8. Click on the *Advanced* tab, press on the *Summary: Residuals & predicted* button. The examined and predicted values of the dependent variable are arranged in the appeared table. The table shows that the predicted and observed values coincide. The model describes the data accurately. Close down the analysis window.

	Predicted & Residual Values (Multi_regression) Dependent variable: pressure/sys								
Case No.	Observed Value	Predicted Value	Residual	Standard Pred. v.	Standard Residual	Std.Err. Pred.Val	Mahalanobis Distance	Deleted Residual	Cook's Distance
Ivanov	145,0000	135,8213	9,17868	-0,10148	1,93640	1,805942	0,680058	10,73727	0,186206
Petrova	127,0000	129,9668	-2,96677	-0,68856	-0,62589	3,715249	5,841025	-7,69261	0,404504
Smirnova	130,0000	128,7014	1,29860	-0,81545	0,27396	2,230899	1,519923	1,66810	0,006858
Koylov	120,0000	118,6475	1,35254	-1,82363	0,28534	3,005156	3,504698	2,26155	0,022874
Orlov	140,0000	140,3142	-0,31422	0,34906	-0,06629	2,220233	1,496680	-0,40254	0,000396
Fedorova	135,0000	135,5149	-0,51486	-0,13221	-0,10862	4,243526	7,899423	-2,59328	0,059972
Stepanova	145,0000	143,3496	1,65044	0,65343	0,34819	2,224922	1,506883	2,11682	0,010985
Belov	150,0000	149,6650	0,33502	1,28672	0,07068	2,383769	1,865293	0,44843	0,000566
Blinov	140,0000	145,6025	-5,60249	0,87935	-1,18194	2,239950	1,539734	-7,21328	0,129283
Adamov	130,0000	136,2677	-6,26765	-0,05673	-1,32227	2,710833	2,681058	-9,31392	0,315697
Ozerov	155,0000	152,1257	2,87431	1,53348	0,60639	2,653537	3,069812	4,50807	0,081950
Pavlov	125,0000	126,0236	-1,02360	-1,08397	-0,21595	2,173153	1,395414	-1,29600	0,003926
Minimum	120,0000	118,6475	-6,26765	-1,82363	-1,32227	1,805942	0,680058	-9,31392	0,000396
Maximum	155,0000	152,1257	9,17868	1,53348	1,93640	4,243526	7,899423	10,73727	0,404504
Mean	136,8333	136,8333	-0,00000	0,00000	-0,00000	2,650597	2,750000	-0,56428	0,101935
Median	137,5000	136,0445	0,01040	-0,07910	0,00219	2,311860	1,702513	0,02295	0,041423

9. Click the *Residuals* tab in the *Residual Analysis* window, set the *Standard residuals* option and press the *Histogram of residuals* button.

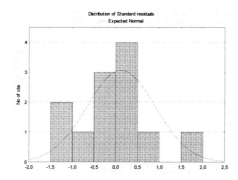

The residuals distribution can be estimated visually as near-normal distribution. It points to a good quality of the model. Close down the histogram.

10.   Click on *Scatterplots* in the *Residual Analysis* window, press the *Residuals vs. deleted residuals* button.

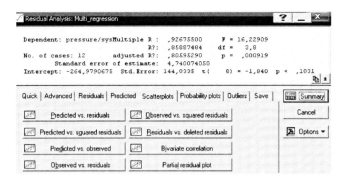

Deleted residuals are a very important statistics which allows one to evaluate the seriousness of the outlying cases problem. These are the standardized residuals for respective observations which one can obtain if the case is excluded from the analysis. Remember that the multiple regression procedure fits the regression surface to express the relations between the dependent and predictor variables. If one case is an outlier (about -3.0 in our case), there is a trend for the regression surface to be pulled by it. As a result, if the respective observation is excluded, another surface will emerge (as well as β-*coefficients*). Therefore, if deleted residuals differ greatly from the standardized residuals, the regression analysis is considered to be seriously biased by the respective observation. In this case the measurement with -3.0 residual going beyond the limits of confidence intervals is the outlier which can affect the analysis. Bur it is a minor outlier as it lies near the dashed line which is the limit of the 95% confidence interval. If the outlier is large, this observation should be deleted.

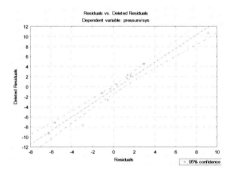

Conclusion: the analysis results have shown that the nonlinear regression model describes the observed values better than the linear model.

Note. *The **GRM (The General Regression Models)** module of the Statistica software package allows developing sophisticated models including plans of effects for categorical predictors. Thus, the word "general" in General Regression Models refers to use of the general linear models. Unlike most other step-by-step regression models, **GRM** is not limited by use of continuous predictors. GRM is an allied module for **GLM (The General Linear Models)**. Both modules use the same methods of analysis and results computing, so that having learnt one module, one can easily get accustomed to another module.*

6.2.3. BINARY LOGISTIC REGRESSION

The binary logistic regression method can be used to investigate the dependence of dichotomous variables from independent ones having any scale type. Consider a specific case. Assume that heart transplant effectiveness is to be predicted. Such kinds of surgeries are very complicated, and there can be only two results: whether a patient is alive or dead (to be more exact, whether a patient is alive the month after the surgery or not- this term is crucial). The pre-surgery data and patient's clinical parameters are age, blood cholesterol level, pressure, blood group, etc. The task comes to the division of the patients into two groups. The forecast for the first group is positive, while for the second group it is negative. It refers to predicting the probability of survival if the dependent variable takes the values *yes* (1) or *no* (0). The solution of this problem can influence the decision to perform a surgery, whether it is worth performing a surgery or not if the probability to stay alive after it is low. The logistic regression is used to predict the probability of some events depending on the predictors values.

Mathematical basis of logit regression

Odds **Odds** = $P/(1 - P)$ are the ratio of the probability that an event will happen to the probability that it will not happen. If one takes a logarithm of probabilities, the obtained expression can be called as *logit*:

$$logit(P) = ln(P/(1 - P)).$$

Let us denote it as y. Then $y = ln(P/(1 - P))$; therefore $P/(1 - P) = e^y$. We determine the probability formula $(e^y \times (1 - P) = P)$ as

$$P = e^y /(1 + e^y).$$

The y variable is called *logit* as it is easy to make this model linear with *logit*. Basically, the *logit regression* is determined by the regression equation $y = a_0 + b_1 x_1 + b_2 x_2 + ... + b_k x_k$. Solving this problem we obtain the values of regression coefficients which will allow one to find the P probability. It is clear that the predicted P values in this model range from 0 to 1 regardless of the regression coefficients or the x values. The odds can be recorded as follows:

$$P/(1 - P) = e^{a_0 + b_1 x_1 + b_2 x_2 + ... + b_k x_k} = e^{a_0}(e^{b_1})^{x_1}...$$

Therefore, if the model with the independent x is correct, the X change per unit leads to the change of the *odds* in e^{b_1} times.

Odds ratio is the ratio of the odds of an event occurring in one group to the odds of it occurring in another group. In terms of logit regression, the odds ratio is understood as the outcome of the simulated odds calculated by the value of the predictor, greater by unity, divided by the odds calculated by the original value of the same predictor. If the e (2.72) number is raised to the power equal to the regression coefficient, we will get the exponential regression coefficient which is interpreted as odds ratio.

In the equation $y = a_0 + b_1 x_1 + b_2 x_2 + ... + b_k x_k$, b_1, b_2 etc. are called the regression coefficients for the risk factors $x_1, x_2, ...$ (age, cholesterol level, etc.) respectively. The axis intercept is denoted as a_0. This is the *value of background risk* which means risk at zero values of all specific risk factors (all x_1, x_2 are equal to zero). Every regression coefficients describes the contribution of corresponding risk factor. Positive regression coefficient means that this factor increases total risk (i.e. increases the analyzed outcome probability), while negative coefficient implies that this factor decreases risk. Large regression coefficient means that the factor influences significantly total risk, while zero regression coefficient denotes the factor having small influence on the outcome probability.

According to this model, the risk (probability) of death as a result of any factors is calculated by the formula:

$$risk\ of\ death = \frac{1}{1 + e^{-y}} = P$$

Perhaps, rising x_2 leads to the increase of the risk of death, but it is quite possible that the risk of death decreases with any other predictor increasing, x_1 as an example.

However, use of logistic transformation in the equation of logit regression causes certain problems. Solving the problem of linear regression, we adjusted a certain hypersurface to the observed values – a line in case of simple regression or a plane in case of two independent variables. Moreover, we required normality and the lack of error correctness. Shifting to the logit regression equation, the surface will not have such a simple form. The normality of errors will not be useful. It makes it impossible to apply the methods of evaluation used in linear problems, the least squares method as an example. Such methods are inapplicable to solve the problems with a large number of predictors. Therefore, the maximum likelihood method is only used to solve the problems of logit regression. The estimation of regression coefficients is limited to maximize the probability of occurrence of a particular sample (at given observed values). Often it leads to low percentage of correct classification rate. Logit regression is weakly stable to excessive adjustment.

Example 6.6. The influence of the spinning room work on the development of upper respiratory airway diseases

Let us assume that you are going to check whether the work experience in the spinning room is connected with the upper respiratory airway diseases or not. Fourteen workers with different work periods (expressed in years) are chosen. Binary response variable takes the value 1 if there is a disease and takes 0 if there are no diseases.

Work order

1. Launch the *Statistica* program. Enter the variables and denote them as *experience* and *diseases*. The initial data look in the following way:

	1 experience	2 diseases
Ivanov	14	0
Petrova	29	1
Smirnova	6	0
Koylov	25	1
Orlov	18	1
Fedorova	4	0
Stepanova	18	0
Belov	12	0
Blinov	22	1
Adamov	6	0
Panin	30	1
Nekrasov	11	0
Antonov	16	1
Zabelin	5	0

The first step in any analysis is understanding of the presented data structure. There is a table with two variables. We suggest a null hypothesis H_0 that the work experience does not influence diseases and an alternative hypothesis H_1 that the work experience in the spinning room is connected with the upper respiratory airway diseases with the level of significance equal to 0.05. Let us look at the work experience distribution among the workers. For this purpose we form a histogram for the *experience* variable.

2. Highlight the *experience* variable and call context menu on right-click. Choose *Graphs of Block Data –Histogram: Entire Columns.*

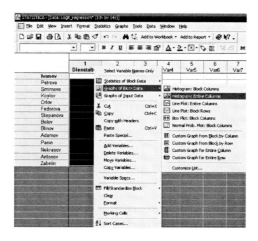

The histogram of the *experience* variable looks in the following way:

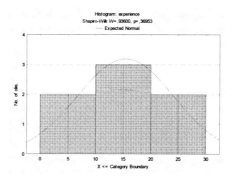

The graph demonstrates that the *experience* variable is uniformly distributed. Let us form a scatterplot to estimate visually the diseases depending on the work experience.

Choose *Graphs –Scatterplots…* in the options menu to display the scatterplot parameter panel.

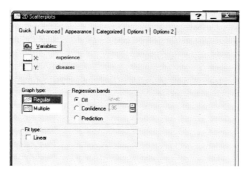

3. Click *Graph type –Regular.* Clear flag from *Linear fit.* Press the *Variables* button. Select the variables to make a scatterplot. Set *experience* as the variable of the *x*-axis and *diseases* as the variable of the *y*-axis. Leave other parameters by default. Press on *OK*.

4. Click on *OK* in the *2D* window to display the scatterplot.

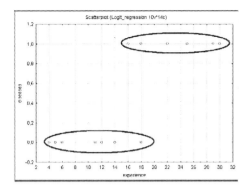

There are two point clouds on the scatterplot. They are encircled by two lines. The first cloud is near the workers with small work experince and without any diseases (opposite to zero), while the second one is next to the workers having with long work experience and some diseases (opposite to one).

5. Choose *Statistics – Advanced Linear/Nonlinear Models – Nonlinear Estimation* in the options menu to make a logit regression model.

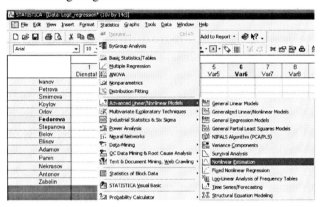

6. Click on *Quick Logit regression* in the appeared *Nonlinear Estimation* window. Press *Ok*.

7. Press on the *Variables* button and choose *Dependent variable – diseases* and *Independent variable list –experience* in the *Logistic Regression* window. Click *OK*.

8. Press Ok in the *Logistic Regression* window.

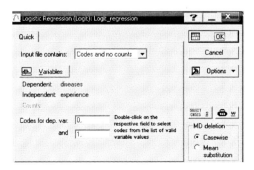

9. The window *Model Estimation* will be displayed where the *Quasi-Newton* estimation method in the *Estimation method* field is set by default. Click on *OK*.

139

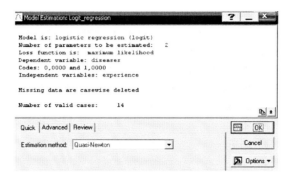

After the calculations the **Results** window will be displayed. The information about the formed model and the estimation results is placed here.

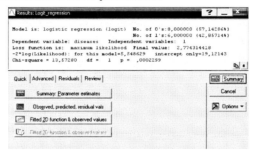

The top of the window has indicated that p-level turned out to be below 5%. The statistic value χ^2/**Chi-square** (13.572) is highly important for the difference between the current model and a model having an absolute term. Therefore, it can be concluded that the work experience is connected with the disease occurrence. The results are arranged in several tables which allow interpreting the results of the regression analysis.

10. Click on the **Quick** tab and the **Summary: Parameter estimates** button to display the analysis table:

	Model: Logistic regression (logit) N of 0's: 8 1's: 6 (Logit_ Dep. var: diseases Loss: Max likelihood Final loss: 2,774314418 Chi?(1)=13,573 p=,00023	
N=14	**Const.B0**	experience
Estimate	-10,9601	1
Odds ratio (unit ch)	0,0000	2
Odds ratio (range)		27175200

The χ^2 criterion takes the value 13.573 in the results table; the level of significance is high. The research results suggest that the length of work experience is closely connected with disease occurrence. The parameters estimates can be interpreted as in the case of standard linear regression model. It means that the absolute term (**Const.B$_0$**)=10.96, and the angular coefficient of the **experience** variable is equal to 2 ($y = -10.96 + 2 \times experience$). However, the estimated parameters refer to the prediction of logit transformation calculated as $y = ln(P/(1 - P))$ and not to the **P** probability determining success or failure. Logit transformation ranges from minus to plus infinity when the values of the P probability lay between 0 and 1. Close the table.

11.   Click on the **Residuals** tab in the **Results** window and press the **Classification of cases & odds ratio** button.

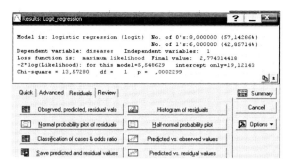

The table with the classification results which allows evaluating the quality of the model will be displayed.

	Classification of Cases (Logit_regression) Odds ratio: 35,000 Perc. correct: 85,71%		
Observed	**Pred. 0,000000**	Pred. 1,000000	Percent Correct
0,000000	7	1	87,50000
1,000000	1	5	83,33334

The table contains the observations which were correctly and incorrectly classified according to the obtained model. For instance, seven out of eight cases were classified correctly as "no", one case was classified as "yes". Five cases out of six were classified as "yes" and one as "no". The prediction probabilities are equal to 87.5% and 83.3%, respectively. This is a good coefficient. The quality of the formed model can be evaluated by the parameter which is called *odds ratio*.

Note. *Odds ratio of a qualified table should not be mixed up with odds ratio of separate predictors, in other words, regression coefficients.*

Odds ratio is calculated as the ratio of the product numbers of correctly classified observations to the product of the misclassified numbers.

Odds ratio which is larger than 1 indicates that the formed classification is better than a random classification. It makes 35 in our example. However, it should be noted that our classification has been chosen to maximize the success probability for the obtained data which corresponded to success. Therefore, if you apply our model to new observations, you should not count on a good classification (as it has already been mentioned, the model is subjected to excessive adjustment).

12. Close the table and return to the **Results** window. Click on the **Quick** tab, choose the option **Observed, predicted, residuals.** It is to be recalled that the regression logit model guarantees that the predicted values will be ranged within the interval [0,1]. Therefore, we can consider the obtained values as probabilities.

	Model is: (Logit_regression) Dep. Var. : diseases		
	Observed	Predicted	**Residuals**
Ivanov	0,000000	0,148960	-0,148960
Petrova	1,000000	0,999706	0,000294
Smirnova	0,000000	0,000902	-0,000902
Koylov	1,000000	0,995927	0,004073
Orlov	1,000000	0,709041	0,290959
Fedorova	0,000000	0,000242	-0,000242
Stepanova	0,000000	0,709041	-0,709041
Belov	0,000000	0,044808	-0,044808
Blinov	1,000000	0,971370	0,028630
Adamov	0,000000	0,000902	-0,000902
Panin	1,000000	0,999848	0,000152
Nekrasov	0,000000	0,023709	-0,023709
Antonov	1,000000	0,395076	0,604924
Zabelin	0,000000	0,000467	-0,000467

13. The prediction rule which the regression logit analysis is based on by default is structured according to the following principle: if the probability $P > 0.5$, we consider that an event will happen, if $P < 0.5$, an event will not happen. The table indicates that in the column of the predicted values named **predicted** six investigated values have the outcome probability "yes"=1 or $P\{y=1\}$ which is more than 0.5. For example, the predicted disease probability for the fifth worker (Avanesov) equals (0.709). Eight workers have the probability value $P\{y=1\}$ which is less than 0.5. This classification rule is optimal in terms of minimizing the number of errors, but it is very rough in terms of the relation research. Often it turns out that the event probability $P\{y=1\}$ is small (significantly lower than 0.5) or great (considerably higher than 0.5). Therefore, it turns out that all combinations of the x variables predict an event, or all of them predict opposite events. For this reason, another classification which demonstrates the relation between dependent and independent variables is required here. Those x_i where $\{y=1\}$ is expected with greater probability on the average are to be referred to the predicted class, while the rest – to the opposite class. In our case a part of the workers fallen ill is equal to $6/14 = 0.43$, and we referred the values for which $P = P\{y = 1\} > 0.43$ to the class of predicted values.

Pressing the **Review** tab displays the results of dotted drawing out with calculated sample parameters.

It is to be mentioned that using the logit regression method, it is necessary to provide a research with other methods, for instance, classification trees. Besides, the **Statistica** package contains the module to carry out the *multinomial logistic regression analysis.* Its results will correlate with the discriminant analysis results which we will consider more particularly.

CHAPTER 7

THE APPLICATION OF STATISTICA SOFTWARE PACKAGE FOR MULTIVARIANCE ANALYSIS

7.1. MULTIVARIATE ANALYSIS OF VARIANCE

Let us consider multivariate analysis of variance based on a hypothetical example. Assume that patients are subjected to three different methods of treatment (***B*1-*B*3** factors); within every method ***A*** factor is divided into four levels (***A*1-*A*4**). The third factor is the age of the patients in the sample divided into three groups: young, middle and old (***C*1-*C*3**). The measurements are performed twice (***R*1-*R*2**). Table 7-1 contains the values of some *hypothetical substance* analysis.

Table 7-1

The initial database for multivariate analysis of variance

Repetitions		*B*1				*B*2				*B*3			
		*A*1	*A*2	*A*3	*A*4	*A*1	*A*2	*A*3	*A*4	*A*1	*A*2	*A*3	*A*4
*R*1	*C*1	26	26	51	104	26	26	51	104	26	26	51	104
*R*1	*C*2	14	86	35	92	14	65	35	92	14	86	35	92
*R*1	*C*3	41	36	96	42	41	36	96	42	41	36	96	42
*R*2	*C*1	16	87	36	133	16	87	36	133	16	87	36	133
*R*2	*C*2	41	39	39	92	41	39	39	92	41	39	39	92
*R*2	*C*3	82	99	114	124	82	73	140	124	82	99	114	124

Work order

1. Launch the ***Statistica*** program.
2. Convert the data from Table 7-1 as the fragment displayed below. Enter the data in 72 lines (6×12) and denote them as ***A*, *B*, *C*** and **Analysis**.

	1 A	2 B	3 C	4 analysis					
1	A1	B1	C1	26	37	A3	B2	C1	51
2	A1	B1	C2	14	38	A3	B2	C2	35
3	A1	B1	C3	41	39	A3	B2	C3	96
4	A1	B1	C1	16	40	A3	B2	C1	36
5	A1	B1	C2	41	41	A3	B2	C2	39
6	A1	B1	C3	82	42	A3	B2	C3	140
7	A2	B1	C1	26	43	A4	B2	C1	104
8	A2	B1	C2	86	44	A4	B2	C2	92
9	A2	B1	C3	36	45	A4	B2	C3	42
10	A2	B1	C1	87	46	A4	B2	C1	133
11	A2	B1	C2	39	47	A4	B2	C2	92
12	A2	B1	C3	99	48	A4	B2	C3	124
13	A3	B1	C1	51	49	A1	B3	C1	26
14	A3	B1	C2	35	50	A1	B3	C2	14
15	A3	B1	C3	96	51	A1	B3	C3	41
16	A3	B1	C1	36	52	A1	B3	C1	16
17	A3	B1	C2	39	53	A1	B3	C2	41
18	A3	B1	C3	114	54	A1	B3	C3	82
19	A4	B1	C1	104	55	A2	B3	C1	26
20	A4	B1	C2	92	56	A2	B3	C2	86
21	A4	B1	C3	42	57	A2	B3	C3	36
22	A4	B1	C1	133	58	A2	B3	C1	87
23	A4	B1	C2	92	59	A2	B3	C2	39
24	A4	B1	C3	124	60	A2	B3	C3	99
25	A1	B2	C1	26	61	A3	B3	C1	51
26	A1	B2	C2	14	62	A3	B3	C2	35
27	A1	B2	C3	41	63	A3	B3	C3	96
28	A1	B2	C1	16	64	A3	B3	C1	36
29	A1	B2	C2	41	65	A3	B3	C2	39
30	A1	B2	C3	82	66	A3	B3	C3	114
31	A2	B2	C1	26	67	A4	B3	C1	104
32	A2	B2	C2	65	68	A4	B3	C2	92
33	A2	B2	C3	36	69	A4	B3	C3	42
34	A2	B2	C1	87	70	A4	B3	C1	133
35	A2	B2	C2	39	71	A4	B3	C2	92
36	A2	B2	C3	73	72	A4	B3	C3	124

3.   Choose *Statistics-ANOVA* in the options menu. Click *Factorial ANOVA-Quick specs dialog* and *OK*.

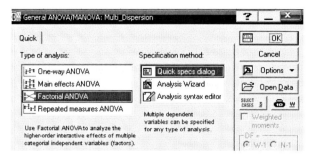

4.   Click on *Variables* in the *ANOVA/MANOVA Factorial ANOVA* window and denote *Dependent variable list -Analysis* and *Categorical predictors (factors)* as *A, B, C*. Press *OK*.

5.   Click *OK*. In the *ANOVA Results* window press *More results* at the bottom of the window.

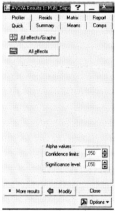

6.   To test the variable distribution, click the tab *Assumptions* in the extended window *ANOVA Results* and choose *A, B, C* effects in the field *Effect*.

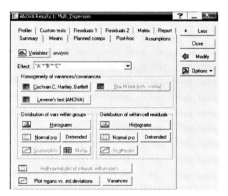

7.   Click *Histograms* in the *Distribution of within-cell residuals* block to display *Residuals* plot. Unfortunately, the *ANOVA* module is not provided with the function of testing the hypothesis about normal distribution with the help of Shapiro-Wilk's or Kolmogorov-Smirnov's

criteria. Visual comparison of the histogram with the red line of normal distribution allows saying that the residuals distribution form is close to normal. It speaks in favor of legitimacy of parametric analysis of variance.

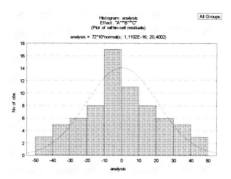

8.   Close the window with the histogram. Choose the **Assumptions** tab in the **ANOVA Results** window to test variance homogeneity, then first of all, denote **A** factor in the **Effect** field and click on the **Levene's test (ANOVA)** button. The displayed table indicates that the significant point 0.084 allows accepting the null hypothesis about variances homogeneity appeared under the influence of **A** factor.

	Levene's Test for Homogeneity of Variances (Multi_C Effect: "A" Degrees of freedom for all F's: 3, 68			
	MS **Effect**	MS Error	F	p
analysis	518,7546	224,7782	2,307851	0,084260

Furthermore, choose **B** and **C** factors from the analysis tables which also indicate the homogeneity of variances.

9.   Return to **ANOVA Results**. Close the analysis tables and click on the **Less** button in order to reduce the number of options. Press the **All effects** button. The results of the general analysis of variance will be displayed. If these results are red, the factor has a significant influence. Analyzing Fisher's criterion and the value of **p-level**, we can say that the outcome of *hypothetical analysis* is influenced by **A, B, C** factors as well as mutual action of two factors **A*C**. The significance level for these factors and **A*C** mutual effect is much lower than the critical level 0.05.

Effect	Univariate Tests of Significance for Analyse (Multi_Dispersion) Sigma-restricted parameterization Effective hypothesis decomposition				
	SS	Degr. of Freedom	MS	F	p
Intercept	297992,0	1	297992,0	363,0605	0,000000
A	34409,4	3	11469,8	13,9743	0,000003
B	12,2	2	6,1	0,0075	0,992567
C	8442,3	2	4221,1	5,1428	0,010649
A*B	308,3	6	51,4	0,0626	0,998900
A*C	20674,6	6	3445,8	4,1982	0,002667
B*C	24,5	4	6,1	0,0075	0,999884
A*B*C	252,6	12	21,1	0,0256	1,000000
Error	29548,0	36	820,8		

10.   Close the analysis window. Click **All effects/Graphs** in the **ANOVA Results** window. The results of the general analysis of variance will be displayed again.

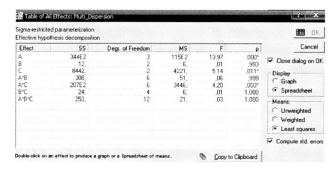

11. Highlight the *A* factor line in the table, set the ***Spreadsheet*** option in the ***Display*** field and click on ***OK***. The table containing the mean values of hypothetical analysis showing the boundaries of the 95% confidence interval in the patients subgroups divided by *A* factor will appear. Close the table and repeat the same procedure with *B* factor, etc. Close the table.

		A; LS Means (Multi_Dispersion) Current effect: F(3, 36)=13,974, p=,00000 Effective hypothesis decomposition				
Cell No.	A	analysis Mean	analysis Std.Err.	analysis -95,00%	analysis +95,00%	N
1	A1	36,66667	6,752686	22,97159	50,3617	18
2	A2	59,55556	6,752686	45,86047	73,2506	18
3	A3	63,27778	6,752686	49,58270	76,9729	18
4	A4	97,83333	6,752686	84,13825	111,5284	18

12. Click the ***More results*** button in the ***ANOVA Results*** window. Press on the ***Summary*** tab and the ***Descriptive cell statistics*** button in the new window.

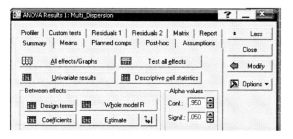

13. The table which fragment is presented below will be displayed. It contains mean values of *Analysis* for different effects including the 95% confidence interval.

					Descriptive Statistics (Multi_Dispersion)				
Effect	Level of Factor	Level of Factor	Level of Factor	N	analysis Mean	analysis Std.Dev.	analysis Std.Err	analysis -95,00%	analysis +95,00%
Total				72	64,3333	36,32250	4,28065	55,798	72,8687
A	A1			18	36,6667	23,56718	5,55484	24,947	48,3863
A	A2			18	59,5556	27,96052	6,59036	45,651	73,4600
A	A3			18	63,2778	35,22667	8,30301	45,760	80,7956
A	A4			18	97,8333	30,13157	7,10208	82,849	112,8174
B	B1			24	64,6250	36,51541	7,45368	49,206	80,0441
B	B2			24	63,7500	37,48884	7,65238	47,920	79,5801
B	B3			24	64,6250	36,51541	7,45368	49,206	80,0441
C	C1			24	59,8750	41,01782	8,37273	42,555	77,1953
C	C2			24	53,8750	28,41664	5,80052	41,876	65,8743
C	C3			24	79,2500	34,86652	7,11710	64,527	93,9728
A*B	A1	B1		6	36,6667	25,08917	10,24261	10,337	62,9961
A*B	A1	B2		6	36,6667	25,08917	10,24261	10,337	62,9961
A*B	A1	B3		6	36,6667	25,08917	10,24261	10,337	62,9961
A*B	A2	B1		6	62,1667	31,84598	13,00107	28,746	95,5870
A*B	A2	B2		6	54,3333	24,09703	9,83757	29,045	79,6216
A*B	A2	B3		6	62,1667	31,84598	13,00107	28,746	95,5870
A*B	A3	B1		6	61,8333	34,39428	14,04141	25,739	97,9279

14. Close down the table and click ***Means*** in the extended the ***ANOVA Results*** window and the first (upper) ***Plot*** button in the ***Plot or show means for effect*** field selecting the de-

sired factor alternately. The plots for the analyzed factors will appear which can help to compare visually the *Analysis* mean values for different effects.

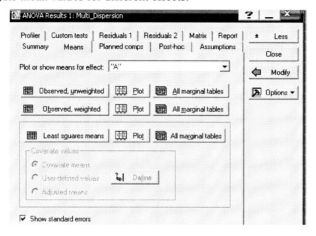

Analysis mean values for different levels of *A* factor

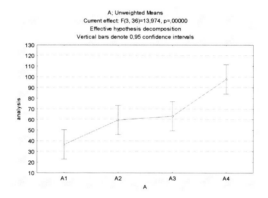

The plot shows that the value of hypothetical analysis increases with growing level of *A* factor. It is clear that the analysis mean value of *A4* level differs from the mean values of other levels. However, it should be checked by statistical tests.

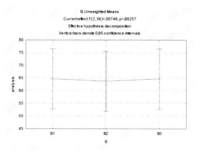

The plot indicates that the *Analysis* mean values of *B* factor at different levels do not differ significantly.

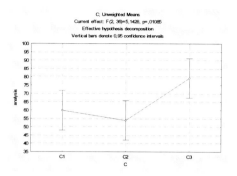

The *Analysis* mean values for various levels of *C* factor are different. The largest value is observed at the third level of the acting *C3* factor (in older age).

15.   Point to the *A* and *C* factors interaction. Select *A* and *C* in *Plot or show means for effect.* Press on *Plot*. Then click *OK* in the appeared *Arrangement of Factors* window.

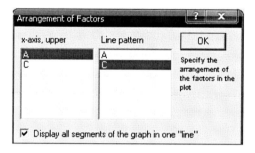

The plot of the *Analysis* mean values in the patients subgroups divided by *A*C* simultaneously will be displayed.

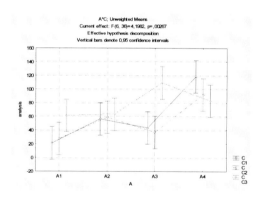

The plot shows that the mean values in some subgroups differ significantly.

16.   In order to find out whether the differences of the means are of a random nature, use the means comparison criteria. Close down the plots window. Click on the *Post-hoc* tab in the *ANOVA Results* window to receive posteriori probabilities. First of all, denote the analyzed *A* factor and choose *Bonferroni* test as the most precise one out of the multiple comparison tests by clicking on the *Bonferroni* button.

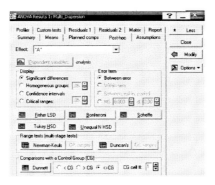

The table where the significance levels below the critical point 0.05 are highlighted in red will appear. If p is less than 0.05, the hypothesis of the means equality is considered to be incorrect, while the alternative hypothesis is correct. In other words, the mean values in the groups are not equal. It is obvious that the statistically significant difference between the mean results of the analysis is observed at the fourth level of the acting A factor towards the first, second and third levels. Close the window.

	Bonferroni test; variable analysis (Multi_Dispersion) Probabilities for Post Hoc Tests Error: Between MS = 820,78, df = 36,000				
Cell No.	A	{1} 36,667	{2} 59,556	{3} 63,278	{4} 97,833
1	A1		0,131128	0,050687	0,000001
2	A2	0,131128		1,000000	0,001766
3	A3	0,050687	1,000000		0,005416
4	A4	0,000001	0,001766	0,005416	

If **Fisher LSD** test is chosen, the results will be quite different. The mean values of the analysis are seen to be different between the first and the second, third and fourth levels; between the second and third as well as between the third and fourth levels. It is connected with less stringency of *Fisher test*.

	LSD test; variable analysis (Multi_Dispersion) Probabilities for Post Hoc Tests Error: Between MS = 820,78, df = 36,000				
Cell No.	A	{1} 36,667	{2} 59,556	{3} 63,278	{4} 97,833
1	A1		0,021855	0,008448	0,000000
2	A2	0,021855		0,699002	0,000294
3	A3	0,008448	0,699002		0,000903
4	A4	0,000000	0,000294	0,000903	

Then choose **B, C** and **A*C** effects one by one to receive the tables based on these factors using **Bonferroni** test.

	Bonferroni test; variable analysis (Multi_Di Probabilities for Post Hoc Tests Error: Between MS = 820,78, df = 36,000			
Cell No.	B	{1} 64,625	{2} 63,750	{3} 64,625
1	B1		1,000000	1,000000
2	B2	1,000000		1,000000
3	B3	1,000000	1,000000	

The mean values of the **B1, B2, B3** subgroups do not differ.

149

	Bonferroni test; variable analysis (Multi_Disp[		
	Probabilities for Post Hoc Tests			
	Error: Between MS = 820,78, df = 36,000			
Cell No.	C	{1} 59,875	{2} 53,875	{3} 79,250
1	C1		1,000000	0,074368
2	C2	1,000000		0,012228
3	C3	0,074368	0,012228	

There are some significant differences of the mean values between the second and the third subgroups under the *C* factor.

Choose *A*C* effect.

Bonferroni test; variable analysis (Multi_Dispersion)
Probabilities for Post Hoc Tests
Error: Between MS = 820,78, df = 36,000

Cell No.	A	C	{1} 21,000	{2} 27,500	{3} 61,500	{4} 56,500	{5} 59,000	{6} 63,167	{7} 43,500	{8} 37,000	{9} 109,33	{10} 118,50	{11} 92,000	{12} 83,000
1	A1	C1		1,000000	1,000000	1,000000	1,000000	1,000000	1,000000	1,000000	0,000349	0,000063	0,008403	0,041181
2	A1	C2	1,000000		1,000000	1,000000	1,000000	1,000000	1,000000	1,000000	0,001164	0,000213	0,026653	0,124017
3	A1	C3	1,000000	1,000000		1,000000	1,000000	1,000000	1,000000	1,000000	0,426203	0,096551	1,000000	1,000000
4	A2	C1	1,000000	1,000000	1,000000		1,000000	1,000000	1,000000	1,000000	0,192240	0,041181	1,000000	1,000000
5	A2	C2	1,000000	1,000000	1,000000	1,000000		1,000000	1,000000	1,000000	0,287508	0,063260	1,000000	1,000000
6	A2	C3	1,000000	1,000000	1,000000	1,000000	1,000000		1,000000	1,000000	0,551207	0,127494	1,000000	1,000000
7	A3	C1	1,000000	1,000000	1,000000	1,000000	1,000000	1,000000		1,000000	0,021087	0,004075	0,384076	1,000000
8	A3	C2	1,000000	1,000000	1,000000	1,000000	1,000000	1,000000	1,000000		0,006609	0,001238	0,134730	0,565431
9	A3	C3	0,000349	0,001164	0,426203	0,192240	0,287508	0,551207	0,021087	0,006609		1,000000	1,000000	1,000000
10	A4	C1	0,000063	0,000213	0,096551	0,041181	0,063260	0,127494	0,004075	0,001238	1,000000		1,000000	1,000000
11	A4	C2	0,008403	0,026653	1,000000	0,041181	1,000000	1,000000	0,384076	0,134730	1,000000	1,000000		1,000000
12	A4	C3	0,041181	0,124017	1,000000	1,000000	1,000000	1,000000	1,000000	0,565431	1,000000	1,000000	1,000000	

Look at the first column *A1*C1*. The differences between $A1^*C1$ with $A3^*C3$, $A1^*C1$ with *A4*C1* subgroups, etc. are statistically important. Close the table.

Note. *The described results of the means comparison in subgroups corresponding to one categorical variable can be obtained using the module Groupings (the difference is only in the criteria of means comparison). To compare the means in subgroups corresponding to the interaction of two or more categorical variables is possible only within the frames of the ANOVA variance module.*

17.	Click the **Summary** tab in the **ANOVA Results** window and press the **Whole model R** button to display the analysis table. It shows that the multiple correlation coefficient is equal to 0.827. The determination coefficient (the fraction of the variance explained) R^2 which equals 0.68 indicates what proportion of variability is explained by the factors under consideration. The table shows that the obtained result is statistically significant p = 0.009377. It can be concluded that the analysis result is influenced by the factors entered into the model. It points to the high quality of the model. Close the window.

Dependnt Variable	Multiple R	Multiple R?	Adjusted R?	SS Model	df Model	MS Model	SS Residual	df Residual	MS Residual	F	p
	Test of SS Whole Model vs. SS Residual (Multi_Dispersion)										
analysis	0,827381	0,684559	0,377880	64124,00	35	1832,114	29548,00	36	820,7778	2,232168	0,009377

18.	Click **Residuals 1** in the **ANOVA Results** window and set the options **Standardized** and **Plot absolute values.**

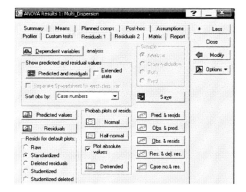

Click on the **Normal** button. The residuals scaterplot is shown in the picture. The correspondence of the variables and their residuals distribution as a whole and in subgroups to the normal distribution law is one of the conditions for use of the parametric analysis of variance. If we identified the model correctly, all the points of the scatterplot would lay close to the line (would be normally distributed). Slight deviations are allowed.

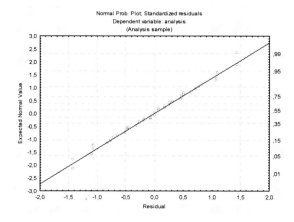

It is obvious that all the residuals lay close to the normal distribution line. It proves the legitimacy of the variance analysis. Close the window.

7.2. CLUSTER ANALYSIS

7.2.1. THE CLASSIFICATION OF THE CLUSTER ANALYSIS METHODS ACCORDING TO CLUSTERING STRATEGIES

The grouping of initial data is the main technique to solve classification problems in applied statistical research. Traditionally, this problem is solved in the following way. The researcher chooses the most informative feature out of a set of features describing the object. The grouping is carried out according to the values of this feature. In multidimensional classification geometric principles are applied. The main concepts of multidimensional analysis are space, its dimensions and relative positions of the objects in this space as well as distances and similarities between them. The similarity of objects is presented by the distance in multidimensional space. It makes it possible to receive more detailed and significant results by investigating the geometric and dynamic features of points' relative positions. In multidimensional **Euclidean** space the distance between two objects is determined by the Pythagorean theorem: the square root of the sum of squares of the differences of the coordinates. $d = \sqrt{\sum (x_i - y_i)^2}$. There are some other concepts in geometry such as *non-Euclidean space* and the multidimensional measurements of space.

Geometric approach in biology and medicine allows investigating various forms of multidimensional variance of biological objects from different angles including morphological and functional characteristics; structure, size and spacial population distribution; the influence of external and internal factors. Those problems which cannot be solved by traditional methods are solved by the methods of multidimensional analysis. For instance, biologists set a goal to separate animals into several kinds to describe the differences between them in detail. According to the modern system applied in biology, a human belongs to primates, mammals, amniotes, vertebrates and animals. In this *classification* the higher the level of aggregation is, the less the similarity between the members of the corresponding class is. A human has more similarities with primates (i.e. apes) than with mammal dogs, etc. In medicine the clustering of diseases, their symptoms and patients according to their health state can be carried out. In psychiatry correct detection of symptoms clusters such as paranoia, schizophrenia, etc. is determining for successful treatment. Computer data processing allows solving time-consuming tasks of multidimensional scaling quickly and easily.

Cluster analysis is a multidimensional method of data analysis. All the elements it contains are similar to each other rather than to the elements of other clusters. Contrary to variance, factor or discriminant analyses, in cluster analysis the requirements of normal distribution to the scale type are not strict. The scale type can influence only the method of clustering, to be more precise, the selection of the required metric space. It would be better to avoid mixed scales. But if it could not be avoided, the following steps are required with mixed scales:
- to apply the method designed for a nominal scale;
- to select a distance measure which is used with mixed scales.

Classically, the clustering of research objects (patients) as well as the clustering of features (symptoms) is carried out simultaneously. But in practice, whether objects or features are chosen. Therefore, the sample of empiric data in multidimensional space is a set of points presented by two different ways:
- a set of points as research objects;
- a set of points as features.

It is the researcher who decides what is more important. In order to carry out clustering, multidimensional feature space is to be turned into metric denoting the method of distance (metric) determination between the points. The function of distance called metric must satisfy many requirements which we will not consider in detail. It is worth mentioning that the concept *Euclidean distance* is widely used for interval or ratio scales, while the concept *Manhattan distance* is applied for nominal and dichotomous scales.

After *metric* space is formed, various methods of clustering are used. The methods are subdivided into *agglomerative* (bottom-up) and *divisive* (top-down). In the first case smaller clusters merge into the larger ones, while in the second case one large cluster is divided into smaller parts. These two processes are carried out until the optimal number of clusters is not obtained. *The maximum number of clusters should not exceed the number of elements in the sample.*

There are three basic methods of clustering analysis implemented in the **Statistica** package:
- agglomerative method which means merging or tree clustering;
- agglomerative method is a two-directional merging based on *objects* (cases) or *variables* (features);
- divisive method which is *K-mean* clustering.

Note. *The results of clustering analysis are the beginning of statistical separation analysis. They cannot be considered to be final and the only possible ones. Opposite conclusions are quite possible in further statistical data processing.*

152

DISTANCE MEASURES IN CLUSTERING ANALYSIS

Euclidean distances. If there is two- or three- dimensional space, it is an ordinary geometric distance between objects in space (as if the distance is measured by a ruler). Usually it is computed from initial data, but not standardized.

City-block (Manhattan) distance. In most cases this distance measure yields results similar to the simple *Euclidean distance*. It is applied when the effect of single large differences (outlying cases) should be dampened.

Chebychev distance metric. This distance measure may be appropriate in the cases when we want to define two objects as *different,* if they are different in one of the coordinates.

Power distance represents only mathematical interest as a universal metric. In some cases it turns into Euclidean or Manhattan distance.

Percent disagreement. This measure is particularly useful if the data are categorical.

All the distances are applicable if the objects of clustering can be presented as k-dimensional space points. The smaller the distance between objects is, the more similar they are.

AMALGAMATION OR LINKAGE RULES

When several objects are linked together, it is necessary to determine **amalgamation or linkage rule** to link two clusters. There are various possibilities:

Nearest neighbour (Single linkage). This method helps to link two clusters when any of the objects in two clusters are closer to each other rather than to corresponding distance linkage. This rule strings objects together to form clusters representing long chains.

Further neighbour (Complete linkage). As an alternative to the first method, *neighbours* in clusters which are further from each other than the rest of the objects pairs can be used.

Unweighted pair-group average. In this method the distance between two clusters is calculated as the average distance between all pairs of objects in two different clusters.

Weighted pair-group average. This method is identical to *the unweighted pair-group average method.* This method should be used when the cluster sizes are suspected to be greatly uneven.

Unweighted pair-group centroid. In this method the distance between two clusters is determined as **the** difference between centroids (average).

Weighted pair-group centroid. This method is identical to the previous one, except that weighting is introduced into the computations in order to take into consideration differences in cluster sizes (i.e. the number of objects contained in them). Therefore, when there are considerable differences in cluster sizes, this method is preferable to the previous one.

Ward's method. This method is distinct from all other methods because it uses the analysis of variance to evaluate the distances between clusters. This method attempts to minimize the Sum of Squares (SS) of any two (hypothetical) clusters that can be formed at every step. The method is regarded as very efficient; however, it tends to create clusters of a small size.

Clustering methods can be subdivided into hierarchical and non-hierarchical. First of all, consider two hierarchical methods.

Agglomeration methods of sample clustering

The purpose of the *agglomeration* type of *joining tree clustering* consists in aggregating objects in larger clusters using the similarity or distance between objects. *Hierarchical tree* which is built in *steps or distance coordinates* is the result of such clustering method. *Horizontal hierarchical tree plot* is presented in the Figure 7.1. In this plot the horizontal axis denotes the *number of steps* in clustering. Steps can be denoted along the vertical axis. The plot starts from every object in class on the left. Before clustering all objects are considered to be separate clusters but they are linked in the algorithm. First, the nearest pair of clusters, which are joined in a common cluster, is chosen. If we gradually (in very small steps) lower the threshold regarding the decision to declare two or more objects to be the members of the same cluster, as a result, we link more and more objects together and aggregate larger and larger clusters consisting of increasingly dissimilar elements. The procedure is repeated until all objects are joined in one cluster. As the Figure shows, there are three clusters at the beginning, then they are linked in the fifth step. Finally, two clusters are left, one of which contains 9 objects, while another one – 5. The clustering is finished in the step 25. The common cluster has formed.

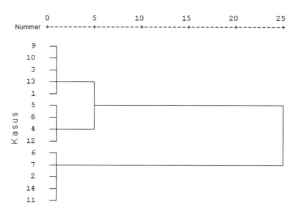

Fig. 7.1 Agglomeration method clustering. Dendrogram construction

Horizontal (or vertical) axes of the second type dendrograms represent distance linkage. For every node in the graph (where a new cluster is formed) we can read off the criterion distance at which the respective elements are linked together into a new single cluster. When the data contain a clear structure of objects similar to each other, then most probably, this structure will be reflected in the hierarchical tree as distinct branches. As the result of a successful analysis with the joining method, we are able to detect clusters (branches) and interpret them.

Two-way joining

Previously, this method was considered in terms of *objects* (cases) or *variables* (features). As an example, the data about different characteristics (variables) of patients' state of health who suffer from pulmonary diseases are collected. The researcher may cluster *cases* (patients) to detect clusters of patients with similar symptoms. At the same time, the researcher may cluster *variables* to detect variables clusters which are connected with similar physical abilities. However, clustering can be carried out *in both directions*. The clustering based on *cases* as well as *variables* can lead to quite interesting results. However, *two-way joining* is used rarely, only in the circumstances when cases and variable are expected to contribute to the uncovering of meaningful patterns of clusters simultaneously. Two-way joining is a rarely applied method because clusters are non-homogeneous in nature. Nevertheless, some researchers believe that this method is a powerful tool for exploratory data analysis.

Divisive method of sample clustering

K – means clustering

This non-hierarchical method of clustering is very different from agglomerative methods of *the joining tree clustering* and *two-way joining*. Different from the hierarchical methods which do not require preliminary assumptions about the number of clusters, in order to use the *k*-mean clustering method it is necessary to have a hypothesis about the most probable number of clusters (in terms of *cases or variables*). In this case *k* of different clusters situated in the larger distance from each other is formed. At first, these points are thought to be the *centers* of the clusters. A *centroid* corresponds to every cluster. Objects are distributed. Furthermore, middle cluster coordinates are counted and new centers are determined. The objects are distributed again. The process of centroids determination and objects distribution continues until the cluster centers are stabilized.

A medical researcher may put forward a hypothesis that generally the patients fall into three different categories (clusters). Then, it is necessary to check whether the hypothesis is confirmed mathematically, whether the *k-means* cluster analysis of the measures of a physical state would produce the three clusters of patients as expected or not. If it is so, the means of the different physical features for each cluster would represent a quantitative way of expressing the researcher's hypothesis (for instance, patients in the first cluster are high on measure 1, but low on measure 2, etc.). As the results of the k-means cluster analysis are obtained, the accuracy of clustering should be tested (in other words, to evaluate how clusters differ from each other). For this purpose all values of the clusters are calculated. In case of accurate clustering the means of all the measures or at least their larger part should differ greatly. The F-statistic values obtained for each measurement is another indicator of how well the respective dimension discriminates between clusters. Computationally, this method can be considered as the *reversed* analysis of variance (ANOVA), as the between group variability is compared with the within-group variability when computing the hypothesis that the means in the groups are different from each other. In *k-means* clustering, the program moves objects (cases) from one cluster to another to get the most significant results. The program starts with k random clusters, and then move objects between those clusters with the goal to minimize variability within clusters and maximize variability *between* clusters to carry out the analysis of variance.

7.2.2. JOINING TREE CLUSTERING

Example 7.1 The severity of herpetic infection
Assume that an immunologist evaluates the severity of herpetic infection. For this purpose the immunologist takes into account damage area and the number of locations on the body in points as well as the rate of recurrence for 24 hours. It is necessary to divide the patients with herpes into 3 groups according to the severity level and compare the results with empirical estimates of the severity provided by the clinician. Later on, we are going to give immune characteristics to the groups and to develop a diagnostic algorithm for classifying patients.

Let us carry out clustering by different methods and compare the results.

Work order

1. Launch the *Statistica* program.
2. Enter the data of 32 cases according to the table and give them corresponding names.

	1 age	2 points	3 quantity of cases
Ivanov	66	6	4
Petrov	40	4	2
Sidorov	50	4	2
Kozlov	70	6	2
Nikulin	54	5	3
Ananin	70	6	3
Rumin	50	5	4
Raikin	49	4	3
Karpov	48	5	3
Skvotzov	70	6	4
Novikov	45	5	3
Aschmann	70	6	3
Afonin	47	5	7
Tarutin	54	5	5
Soloviev	49	5	7
Sizov	48	5	7
Vanin	50	5	4
Logvin	52	5	3
Pronin	48	5	3
Filin	47	5	4
Kuklin	48	5	3
Pronin	70	7	4
Lubschin	50	5	4
Frolov	54	5	5
Laboda	60	4	5
Rumin	70	7	4
Nosov	50	4	5
Udatschin	48	5	4
Fomin	51	5	3
Sanaev	52	4	5
Zizin	47	5	7
Gromov	51	5	4

The variable are different in scale; therefore they should be standardized.
3. Choose *Data-Standardize* the options menu.

155

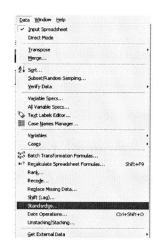

4. Click the *Variables* button in the *Standardization* window and set 1-3; *Cases* are left by default – All; *weight* is not set.

The window will look in the following way:

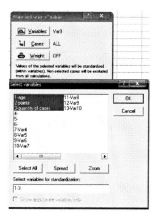

5. Press *OK*. The variable will range from -1 to 1. The mean is subtracted from the values of the variables. These values are divided by standard deviation *(Z-Scores)*.

	1 age	2 points	3 quantity of cases
Ivanov	1,342724	1,166247	-0,0219264505
Petrov	-1,56651	-1,40754	-1,42521928
Sidorov	-0,44757	-1,40754	-1,42521928
Kozlov	1,790299	1,166247	-1,42521928
Nikulin	0	-0,12065	-0,723572866
Ananin	1,790299	1,166247	-0,723572866
Rumin	-0,44757	-0,12065	-0,0219264505
Raikin	-0,55947	-1,40754	-0,723572866
Karpov	-0,67136	-0,12065	-0,723572866
Skvotzov	1,790299	1,166247	-0,0219264505
Novikov	-1,00704	-0,12065	-0,723572866

6. Choose *Multivariate Exploratory Techniques-Cluster Analysis* in the options menu.

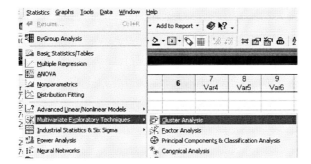

The displayed window contains three methods.

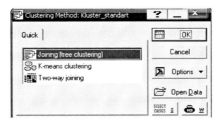

7. Click ***Joining (tree clustering)*** and press ***OK***.

8. The ***Cluster analysis*** window will be displayed. Select the ***Advanced*** tab, click the ***Variables*** button and set three variables for the analysis. Press on ***OK***.

9. There is the ***Raw data*** type in the ***Input file*** field of the ***Cluster analysis*** window as the data have just been entered. Previously saved file may also be opened.

The direction of the classification is set in the ***Cluster*** field. In this case ***Cases-rows*** are to be marked. While clustering the variables, ***Variables-Columns*** are marked.

The ***Amalgamation (linkage) rule*** line contains the settings to select different similarity measures. For this case choose ***Ward's method.***

Different distance types are presented in the ***Distance measure*** window.

Click on ***City-block (Manhattan) distance.***

Go to the ***MD (Missing data) deletion*** line.

The Statistica system in the ***Cluster Analysis*** module provides two ways to process incomplete observations containing the gap of at least one variable:

• ***Casewise deleted*** are incomplete observations which are excluded from the further analysis. However, this method leads to bias and inconsistency of the statistical estimates as well as to a distortion of the empirical distribution.

• ***Substituted by means*** is the way when missing data are replaced by the mean values obtained from the complete (complex) data, which also has its drawbacks.

In this case choose ***Casewise***. As a result, the window will be displayed in the following way:

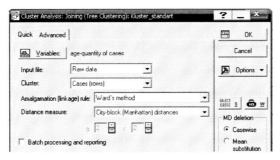

10. Click **OK** to see the **Joining Results** window. Press the **Advanced** tab.

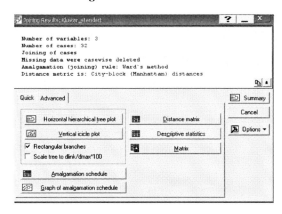

11. To visualize clustering analysis press the **Vertical icicle plot** button. The horizontal axis of the dendrogram represents *observations*, while vertical – *linkage distance*. The linking process is observed. There are three clusters at the distance equal to 13. While increasing the distance up to 15, the number of clusters makes 2. There is only one cluster at the distance equal to 38.

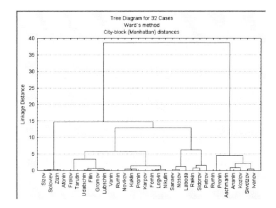

12. Close the window. Press the **Advanced** tab in the **Joining Results** window and click on the **Amalgamation schedule** button to display the table of the results with the linkage scheme. The first column contains the distances of the corresponding clusters. Every line indicates the cluster's contents at this step of classification. For instance, Ananin and Aschmarin are united at the first step (the first line), Rumin and Vanin – at the second step (the second line), Rumin, Vanin, Lubshin – at the third step (the third line), Karpov, Pronin – at the fourth step (the fourth line), etc. The linkage is finished at 38.7.

linkage distance	Obj. No. 1	Obj. No. 2	Obj. No. 3	Obj. No. 4	Obj. No. 5	Obj. No. 6	Obj. No. 7	Obj. No. 8	Obj. No. 9
Amalgamation Schedule (Kluster_standart) Ward's method City-block (Manhattan) distances									
0,000000	Ananin	Aschmarin							
0,000000	Rumin	Vanin							
0,000000	Rumin	Vanin	Lubschin						
0,000000	Karpov	Pronin							
0,000000	Karpov	Pronin	Kuklin						
0,000000	Afonin	Zizin							
0,000000	Tarutin	Frolov							
0,000000	Pronin	Rumin							
,1118937	Logvin	Fomin							
,1118937	Soloviev	Sizov							
,1118937	Filin	Udatschin							
,1678405	Rumin	Vanin	Lubschin	Gromov					
,2237873	Nosov	Sanaev							
,2797342	Afonin	Zizin	Soloviev	Sizov					
,3356810	Nikulin	Logvin	Fomin						
,4475747	Ivanov	Skvotzov							
,5035215	Karpov	Pronin	Kuklin	Novikov					
,6900110	Rumin	Vanin	Lubschin	Gromov		Filin	Udatschin		
,8135401	Sidorov	Raikin							
,9355286	Kozlov	Ananin	Aschmarin						
1,268128	Laboda	Nosov	Sanaev						
1,478595	Nikulin	Logvin	Fomin	Karpov	Pronin	Kuklin	Novikov		
1,613904	Petrov	Sidorov	Raikin						
2,139602	Ivanov	Skvotzov	Kozlov	Ananin	Aschmarin				

13. Close the table. Click the ***Advanced*** tab in the ***Joining results*** table. Press ***Graph of amalgamation schedule*** and look through the results of tree clustering. The horizontal axis indicates steps, the vertical axis – distances. The total amount of steps to link all the objects into one cluster constitutes 30.

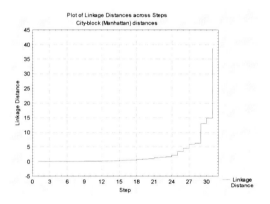

14. Close the plot. Click the ***Distance matrix*** button in the ***Advanced*** tab in the window with the classification results ***(Joining Results)*** which is saved by the option ***Save distance matrix*** for further analysis. ***City-block (Manhattan) distance*** will appear between different cases (patients).

Case No.	Ivanov	Petrov	Sidorov	Kozlov	Nikulin	Ananin	Rumin	Raikin	Karpov	Skvotzov	Novikov
Ivanov	0,00	6,89	5,77	1,85	3,33	1,15	3,08	5,18	4,00	0,45	4,3
Petrov	6,89	0,00	1,12	5,93	3,56	6,63	3,81	1,71	2,88	7,33	2,5
Sidorov	5,77	1,12	0,00	4,81	2,44	5,51	2,69	0,81	2,21	6,21	2,5
Kozlov	1,85	5,93	4,81	0,00	3,78	0,70	4,93	5,63	4,45	1,40	4,7
Nikulin	3,33	3,56	2,44	3,78	0,00	3,08	1,15	1,85	0,67	3,78	1,0
Ananin	1,15	6,63	5,51	0,70	3,08	0,00	4,23	4,92	3,75	0,70	4,0
Rumin	3,08	3,81	2,69	4,93	1,15	4,23	0,00	2,10	0,93	3,52	1,2
Raikin	5,18	1,71	0,81	5,63	1,85	4,92	2,10	0,00	1,40	5,63	1,7
Karpov	4,00	2,88	2,21	4,45	0,67	3,75	0,93	1,40	0,00	4,45	0,3
Skvotzov	0,45	7,33	6,21	1,40	3,78	0,70	3,52	5,63	4,45	0,00	4,7
Novikov	4,34	2,55	2,55	4,79	1,01	4,08	1,26	1,73	0,34	4,79	0,0
Aschmarin	1,15	6,63	5,51	0,70	3,08	0,00	4,23	4,92	3,75	0,70	4,0
Afonin	5,52	5,58	5,13	7,37	3,59	6,67	2,44	4,32	2,92	5,97	3,0

7.2.3. DIVISIVE CLUSTERING BY K-MEANS METHOD

Let us consider the example 7.1
Work order
1. Choose *Multivariate Exploratory Techniques-Cluster Analysis.*
2. Click *K-means clustering* in a new *Clustering Method* and press *OK.*

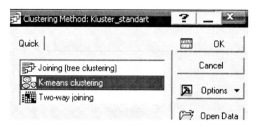

3. The *Cluster analysis:K-means* window will be displayed. Click *Advanced,* press *Variables* and denote three variables. Click *OK.*

4. Press *Gases (rows)*; *Number of clusters* in the *Cluster* field. Denote three, at first. Then, denote the maximum number of iterations (recomputation) 10 (from 5 to 99 is possible), otherwise the procedure may get stuck.

The set of options *Initial cluster centres* is important while changing the parameters as the final results depend on the initial configuration.

The *Choose observations to maximize initial between-cluster distances* option selects the first *k* observations (according to a number of clusters) which serve as the centres of clusters. Further observations substitute the chosen centres if the least distance up to any object is more than the least distance between clusters. As a result of this procedure, the initial distances between clusters are maximized.

If the *Sort distances and take observations at constant intervals* option is chosen, firstly, the distances between objects are sorted out, then the observations at regular intervals are taken as initial centres of clusters.

The *Choose the first N (Number of cluster) observation* option takes the first *N* cluster observations as initial centres. For our example set *Sort distances and take observations at constant intervals.*

In the group of options *MD deletion* leave *Casewise.*

If the *Batch processing and reporting* option is set, the *Statistica* system will conduct a complete analysis automatically and present the results according to the settings. Click *OK.*

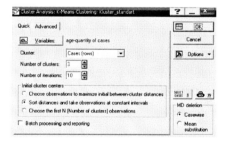

5. Choose the *Advanced* tab in the appeared *k-means Klustering Results* window.

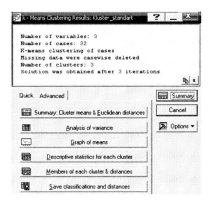

6. Click the ***Graph of means*** button to see the mean value of every cluster in the graph. It indicates that the greater difference is between the clusters 1 and 2. The points of their mean values for three parameters have the largest distance from each other.

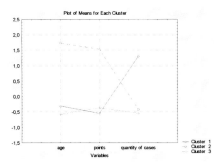

7. Close the graph. Click ***Summary: Cluster means & Euclidean distances*** to display the table which indicates the distances from each cluster to other two clusters below zeros. The squared distances are placed above zeros. The greater the distance is, the more different the clusters are. It is shown that the largest distance 1.955 is between the clusters 1 and 2. Its square is equal to 3.823. Close the window.

Cluster Number	Euclidean Distances between Clusters (Kluster_ Distances below diagonal Squared distances above diagonal		
	No. 1	No. 2	No. 3
No. 1	0,000000	3,823748	1,178741
No. 2	1,955441	0,000000	2,977127
No. 3	1,085698	1,725435	0,000000

8. Click on ***Descriptive statistics for each cluster*** to display three tables for each analysis. For instance, in the third cluster the mean (standardized) value of ***Age*** is -0.580448, ***Points*** is -0.361939 and ***Quantity*** is -0.548161. Close the window.

	Descriptive Statistics for Cluster 3 (Kluster_standar Cluster contains 16 cases		
Variable	Mean	Standard Deviation	**Variance**
age	-0,580448	0,354355	0,125567
points	-0,361939	0,518763	0,269115
quantity of cases	-0,548161	0,479316	0,229744

161

9. Click the *Members of each cluster & distances* button to display the window with three tables for different clusters and with the contained elements indicating the standardized distance. 16 cases are aggregated in the cluster 3. Karpov has the least distance to the cluster's center (0.180052), while Petrov has the largest distance (0.97).The first one can be called as the typical representative of the cluster, and the second is the least typical one. Close the window.

>k5* ter Analysis (Kluster_standart) K-means clustering results dialog	Members of Cluster Number 3 (Kluster and Distances from Respective Cluster Cluster contains 16 cases
Members of Cluster Number 1 (Kluster_stand Members of Cluster Number 2 (Kluster_stand Members of Cluster Number 3 (Kluster_stand	Distance
Petrov	0,972082
Sidorov	0,791668
Nikulin	0,376790
Rumin	0,342929
Raikin	0,612234
Karpov	0,180052
Novikov	0,300541
Vanin	0,342929
Logvin	0,268451
Pronin	0,180052
Filin	0,354154
Kuklin	0,180052
Lubschin	0,342929
Udatschin	0,336334
Fomin	0,222787
Gromov	0,362885

10. Click the *Analysis of variance* button. The analysis of variance table compares the value of between-group and intra-variances. The lower the value of intra-variance compared to the between-group is, the more accurate clustering has become. The results of variance analysis have shown that the separation has been successful, as the *p* level of significance at Fisher's criterion is less than 0.05 for all variables. The variables with $p>0.05$ are excluded from the clustering procedure. Close the window of variance analysis.

	Analysis of Variance (Kluster_standart)					
Variable	Between SS	df	Within SS	df	F	signif. p
age	27,12240	2	3,877596	29	101,4223	0,000000
points	21,28524	2	9,714764	29	31,7698	0,000000
quantity of cases	21,34921	2	9,650795	29	32,0765	0,000000

11. Press the *Save classifications and distances* button. Choose three analyzed variables in the window foe selection. Click on *OK* to see the analysis table.

	Kluster_standart					
	1 age	2 points	quantity of	4 CASE_NO	5 CLUSTER	6 DISTANC
Ivanov	1,342724	1,166247	-0,0219264505	1	2	0,38
Petrov	-1,56651	-1,40754	-1,42521928	2	3	0,97
Sidorov	-0,44757	-1,40754	-1,42521928	3	3	0,79
Kozlov	1,790299	1,166247	-1,42521928	4	2	0,62
Nikulin	0	-0,12065	-0,723572866	5	3	0,38
Ananin	1,790299	1,166247	-0,723572866	6	2	0,28
Rumin	-0,44757	-0,12065	-0,0219264505	7	3	0,34
Raikin	-0,55947	-1,40754	-0,723572866	8	3	0,61
Karpov	-0,67136	-0,12065	-0,723572866	9	3	0,18
Skvotzov	1,790299	1,166247	-0,0219264505	10	2	0,32
Novikov	-1,00704	-0,12065	-0,723572866	11	3	0,30

Analyzing the displayed information, it can be concluded that this sample is worth dividing into three clusters, but the division into two or four clusters is not excluded. Everything depends on the situation and the researcher. Repeat the clustering procedure having excluded the variable *Age*. Draw the conclusions.

The module provides the ability to save the clustering results for further investigations. Each observation in a new file is assigned to the number of the cluster which it belongs to in the classification (the column *Cluster*) and the distance to the corresponding cluster (the column *Distance*).

The **Tables and banners** module allows checking whether the distribution of patients in groups according to the severity level and the number of relapses per year provided by the immunologist coincides with the clustering analysis results or not. For this purpose click the **Statistics-Basic Statistics-Tables- Tables and banners-Advanced-Members of each cluster & distances** division. Compare two distributions and draw the conclusions about the clustering success.

Conclusions. *The considered methods of medical data classification allowed formulating diagnostics rules where experts find it difficult to formalize their knowledge and create a comprehensive classification model. The obtained algorithm requires no calculations. It can be carried out directly at the patient's admission and it is a convenient and reliable enough method for practical use.*

7.3. FACTOR ANALYSIS

7.3.1. BASIC CONCEPTS OF FACTOR ANALYSIS

Factor analysis originated in the intelligence study in psychology. Francis Galton formulated the first principles. *Factor analysis is a set of statistical models describing and explaining observed variables in terms of a lower number of unobserved (latent) factors which can be constructed by definite mathematical methods.* The detection of latent factors is based on the assumption that if several signs measured in a group change concordantly, we assume the existence of a latent common cause of the joint variability.

As far as *factor* is interpreted as the cause of the joint variability of several initial variables, then the factor analysis, in fact, is the correlation analysis of a set of attributes. It is based on such statistical concepts as a mean value, variance, correlation, co-variance and is applied in solving the following problems:
- to reduce the number of variables (data reduction);
- to detect structure in the relationships between variables that is to classify variables;
- to convert initial variables to be more convenient to visualize or interpret;
- to interpret indirect factors which are not measured directly.

The factor analysis model is the original variables presentation as a linear combination of the **F** factors where the relationship between the features and factors is defined.

There are two models of factor analysis:

1) a model of the *actual* factor analysis when the observed values are determined not only by factors, but by the influence of local and accidental causes according to the following law:

$$X_i = \sum_{j=1}^{k} a_{ij} F_j + b_i U_i$$

The variables F_j called as *common factors* and constant coefficients a_{ij} called as *factor loadings* (the loading of *i*-variable on *j*-factor) are unknown parameters to be estimated where $j = 1, 2,\ldots, k$, $i=1, 2, \ldots, n$. *Factor loadings* are analogous to the correlation coefficients. The greater the absolute value of the load factor is, the stronger the relation of the variable with the factor is and the more the variable is determined by this factor. The variables $Ui, i = 1, 2,\ldots,n$ are known as unique factors influenced by local accidental causes.

2) the method of principle components in which main components F_j called *common factors* are connected with the observed variables X_i by linear transformation function in the following way:

$$X_i = \sum_{j=1}^{k} a_{ij} F_j$$

Thus, the method of principle components can be considered as a special case of factor analysis when all unique factors are equal to zero. This chapter is not aimed at the detailed description of differences between the methods of *principle components* and *factors*. It requires the understanding of complex mathematical techniques. It should be noted that despite the differences, these methods have similar solution algorithm. Let us pay attention to the principle parameters of factor analysis.

Assume that four features which are influenced by two factors F_1 and F_2 are measured in the research. The factor F_1 influences four characteristic features of the object, while F_2 deals only with two features X_2 and X_3.

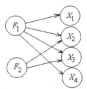

Fig. 7.2

Thus, the values of the X_1 and X_4 features are determined only by the F_1 factor. The X_2 and X_3 features are defined by the joint effects of the F_1 and F_2 factors. As it is unknown, we are aimed at estimating the intensity of the factors F_1 and F_2 impact on the X_i features and at marking those X_i values which are influenced by each of the F_1 and F_2 factors separately.

The method which allows reflecting the properties of dozens of indicators in a single factor makes it possible to compare only a few components rather than many indicators of a system with other parameters. Based on the group composition, every factor can be interpreted. In other words, we can describe the properties of a factor with corresponding adjectives (hormonal, hematological, humoral, etc.).

The required conditions of factor analysis are:
- All features are to be quantitative.
- The number of observations should be twice as the number of variables.
- The sample should be homogeneous.
- The initial variables are to be distributed simultaneously.
- Factor analysis is carried out according to correlated variables.

Bartlett's test is used to check the hypothesis about multivariate normal distribution as a whole. It is difficult to test this hypothesis in practice; therefore, factor analysis is applied without such kind of procedure. Moreover, some researchers consider this assumption unnecessary.

Stages of factor analysis:
- Selection of factors for the analysis of the observed parameters. Here, the number of factors is considerably smaller than the number of the original variables.
- Classification and systematization of factors.
- Modelling of correlation between resultative and factorial variables.
- Estimation of factorial influence and evaluation of their roles in the change of resultative variable.
- Factor model operation (its practical use).

In factor analysis evaluation procedure includes:
- Evaluation of the factor structure and determination of the optimal number of factors;
- Evaluation of the factor loading and determination of the optimal number of variables included into this factor;
- Interpretation of factors.

Main indicators of factor analysis

Component matrix reflects the factor structure. It consists of factor loadings; its number of columns equals to the number of common factors, and the number of rows equals to the number of original features. Matrix is built by reducing the number of variables while their maximum variance is maintained where the total variance of each variable is divided into components.

In component matrix *factor loadings* are the separate elements of matrix that reflect the degree of correlation between corresponding variables and factors. They are the equivalents of correlation coefficient which vary from -1 to +1. The larger their value is, the stronger the correlation between the variable and factor is, and the more this variable is associated with the influence of the corresponding factor. It is important that each variable must have factor loadings close to zero (not larger than 0.2) in every factor except for one. The sum of the squares of the factor loadings of all factors equals to the total variance or the sum of the eigenvalues.

Communality is a part of the variance of variable which is explained by all factors or a couple of them. Total variance consists of two terms, namely *explained variance* H_i^2 and the variance of a specific factor $S_{U_i}^2$, so called specificity, associated with accidental mistakes or the variables that were not taken into account in the model.

Variance of the feature = Communality + Specificity

While analyzing, it is necessary to find such factors using which the total communality is maximum, and the specificity is minimum. It is desirable that all emphasized factors explain 80% of the scatter. If the value of communality is smaller than the threshold value, it is recommended to reduce the number of features or increase the number of factors. The sum of the squares of factor loadings for each factor in all features (in a column) reflects its contribution to the total variance of the systematized features. So, the greater this contribution is, the more important this factor is.

The sum of the squares of the factor loadings of i-feature to the full set of factors (according to a row) equals to the total variance of the variable explained by all factors. Factors are ranged in descending order of their variances.

Eigenvalue is an index taken as the capacity of a factor. It is estimated as the sum of the squares of the factor loadings *in a column*. The eigenvalues of the factors are singled out in the decreasing order. The larger the correlation between the initial variables is, the greater the previous eigenvalues are, and the smaller the following ones are. The number obtained by dividing the eigenvalue factor on the total number of variables is interpreted as the fraction of variance explained by this component.

The essence of factor analysis is a procedure called factor rotation. This procedure is used to convert the structure of factors obtained on the previous stage into the simpler and more obvious one. It is reached by repartitioning the variance using a certain method obtained as a result of several iterates. There are various kinds of rotation, such as:
- *Varimax* and *Varimax normalized*;
- *Biquartimax*;
- *Quartimax*;
- *Equamax*.

The choice of the rotation method usually depends on the set objectives. Here, different criteria of rotation are used. Often simple structure is used as a criterion for rotation according to the following rule: the maximum value of a variable is reached according to one factor, and the minimum one is reached according to the rest factors. If rotation does not make any important changes in the structure of the factor space, it proves the stability of both rotation and data. In analysis the variables that have strong correlation between each other are joined into one factor, and as a result the variance between components is repartitioned, and we obtain simpler and more reasonable factor structure. After joining the correlation between the components inside each factor will be greater than between the components of other factors. This procedure also allows us to single out hidden latent variables.

Evaluation of factor loadings may be realized with the help of different methods, such as:
- *Principal components*;
- *Principal factor*;
- *Principal axis method*;
- *Maximum likelihood factors*;
- *Centroid method*.

7.3.2. PRINCIPAL COMPONENTS METHOD

This method transforms the set of correlating initial variables into another set of non-correlating variables. As the result of transformations, we find such an axis (principal component) for correlating variables along which we see the maximum variance (**Varimax**) of the objects which means that the amount of the data is maximum. When passing from the initial coordinate system to the new one, some portion of information may be lost; however, at the same time, dimensionality is reduced. The stronger the correlation between variables is, the smaller portion of information about them is lost.

To define the *optimum quantity of factors* three criteria can be applied.

The main criterion in making decision about the number of factors is explained variance. It is recommended to single out such number of factors that cumulative percent of explained by them variance exceeds 80%. For example, if percent of total variance explained by the first factor equals to 47%, and percent of total variance explained by the second factor is 35%, two factors should be singled out, as their cumulative percent exceeds 80%.

The second criterion is called the Kaiser criterion, and it suggests that the eigenvalues must be larger than 1.

Finally, the third criterion is called the Cattell criterion or the inflection point on the scree plot. The data under observation may be depicted as a scree plot. The divisions along the horizontal axis are the number of factors before rotation (the number of eigenvalues), and its vertical axis corresponds to eigenvalues. At first, (*number of eigenvalues* =1, 2,...) the eigenvalues decrease quickly (sharp decline of the plot), but then (usually when *number of eigenvalues* =3, 4,...) decrease of eigenvalues becomes slower. If this deceleration is sharp (on some certain factor number), its point of the sharp fall of the slope is called the inflection point of the plot. It is recommended to single out the number of factors which corresponds to the sharp part of the plot. If the plot does not have the sharp inflection, the criterion of the inflection is not taken into account. If there is the inflection point, we look at the situation. For instance, if the plot inflection occurs in case of eigenvalues which are close to 1, the criterion of the scree plot is preferential. If the plot inflection occurs when the eigenvalues are very small, the criteria 'eigenvalues>1' and 'explained variance>80%' are preferential.

The variable is included in factor, if it has the largest loading. On default the program highlights the loadings exceeding 0.7 in modulus. Let us consider the loading 0.7 as a borderline. If the loading exceeds 0.7, the variable is included in factor; if the loading does not exceed 0.7, the variable is not included in factor. However, it is not necessarily 0.7 that must be a borderline, it is just a recommendation. In any case, if the loading is just a little bit different from 0.7, we can include such variable in factor.

Example 7.2.

It is considered that not only nutritional habits (the amount of fat in food, for example), but also some anthropo-constitutive parameters influence the prevalence of hormone-dependent malign neoplasms. Assume that there is a group of examined patients whose ten hypothetic parameters (height, weight, and hormones level) evaluated in points (in interval scale) were measured. It is required to find the main factors influencing the state of health and find out possible correlation between them.

Table 7-3

The initial data for factor analysis

№	X1	X2	X3	X4	X5	X6	X7	X8	X9	X10
Ivanov	3	4	3	4	7	8	7	6	8	7
Petrov	5	5	5	4	6	5	6	3	4	3
Sidorov	3	4	3	3	4	5	5	5	4	5
Kozlov	3	4	3	3	5	5	4	7	6	7
Nikulin	6	7	6	7	8	7	7	7	8	8
Ananin	7	6	5	6	4	5	4	5	4	5
Rumin	4	4	4	4	5	6	6	7	6	5
Raikin	6	5	5	5	5	4	4	6	5	5
Karpov	5	5	5	6	7	6	6	3	4	4
Skvotzov	5	5	4	5	6	5	6	6	5	5
Novikov	4	4	5	4	4	3	4	3	4	4
Aschmarin	5	6	5	5	5	4	5	5	5	5
Afonin	5	4	5	5	5	6	5	5	5	5
Tarutin	5	5	4	5	4	3	4	5	3	4
Soloviev	5	6	5	5	6	7	7	6	5	5
Sizov	8	7	8	7	8	9	8	5	5	5
Vanin	4	5	3	4	4	4	4	6	7	7
Logvin	3	4	5	4	5	4	6	5	5	5
Pronin	4	5	4	4	5	6	5	6	7	6
Filin	5	5	6	5	5	4	5	4	3	4
Kuklin	5	4	5	4	5	6	5	4	5
Pronin	5	5	6	4	5	5	4	6	5	6
Lubschin	6	7	9	6	5	5	6	5	5	5
Frolov	4	4	4	4	5	5	5	4	5	5
Laboda	5	5	6	4	4	5	5	6	5	5

Work order

1.   Launch the **Statistica program**. Insert the data. In operational menu choose **Multivariate exploratory techniques – Factor analysis**.

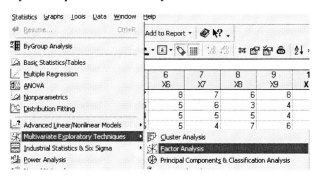

2.   Then, in **Factor Analysis** window in **Input file** field set – **Raw Data**. Switch on **MD deletion – Casewise**. Due to this option in the electronic spreadsheet containing the data, the rows (cases) that have at least one missed value are ignored. Press the **Variables** button. Set the variables from 1 to 10 with the help of the mouse or the **Select All** button. Press **Ok**.

3.   The *Define Method of Factor Extraction* window will be displayed. Choose the *Advanced* tab.

In the upper part of the window the following data is displayed: missed data is processed with the help of **Casewise** method **(missed cases-lines are deleted)** – 25 out of 25 cases are processed and taken for the further estimation; correlation matrix is estimated for 10 variables.

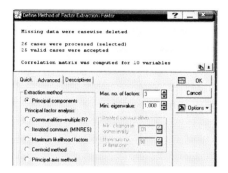

The bottom part of the window contains the options for choosing the method, and the field in which settings for iterative calculation of the communalities are conducted.

In the right part of the window there are the ***Maximum no. of factors*** field that defines the number of factors that will be highlighted by the system, and the ***Minimum eigenvalue*** field in which the values which are smaller than the one set in the field are ignored.

The group of options united under the name ***Extraction method*** allows us to choose the way of procession. Depending on the criterion of optimality, the analysis is possible either with the help of **principal components** or one of the methods united in the **Principal factor analysis** group.

4.   Set the maximum number of factors that equals to 3. Leave the ***Min. Eigenvalues*** field to be equal to 1 on default. Set the **Principal Components** option. Press **Ok**. The *Factor Analysis:Resylts* window of analysis will be displayed. Choose the **Loadings** tag.

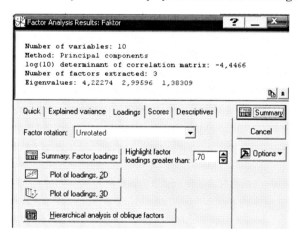

In the upper part of this window the data message is given:
- Number of variables: 10;
- Method: Principal components;
- Log(10) of determination of correlation matrix: - 4.4466
- Number of factor extraction: 3; Eigenvalues: 4.22274; 2.99596 and 1.38309.

The ***Factor rotation*** option helps us to choose various rotations of axes, i.e. to rotate the factors to find the optimal solution. The rotation is aimed at maximization of variability of a new variable and minimization of original variable dispersion.

The following ways of rotation are possible: **Biquartimax; Quartimax; Equamax**.

The additional term in the name is **'normalized'** that shows that factor loadings are normalized in the procedure, i.e. they are divided by the square root of the corresponding communalities; and also the term **'raw'** is used, and it refers to the initial type of data showing that the rotated loadings are not normalized.

In the bottom part of the window there are tags and functional buttons that allows us to look through the analysis results both numerically and graphically.

5.   In the **Factor rotation** field leave the **Unrotated** factor loadings, and press the **Plot of Loadings 3D** button. It is possible to look at the results of factor analysis on the plot. Here, the variables that are included in each of three factors may be observed. If the number of factors and variables included in these factors are chosen correctly, the groups of variables included in these factors are densely placed in the diametrically opposite parts of the space. Close the plot window.

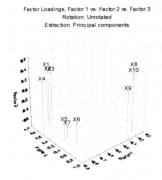

Factor Loadings, Factor 1 vs. Factor 2 vs. Factor 3
Rotation: Unrotated
Extraction: Principal components

6.   Press the **Summary: Factor loading** button. The table that contains the correlation coefficients of variables and highlighted factors will be displayed. Significant loadings that are greater than 0.7 are highlighted red. It is seen from the plot that three vectors are likely to be significant, and factor loadings display two vectors. It makes interpretation complicated. When analyzing such table, it is better to exclude the factor that does not have maximum loading of variable, and also those variables that does not have the same high loadings in two or more factors. However, it leads to missing data. In such cases it is better to use the rotation of axes to obtain an optimal solution.

Variable	Factor Loadings (Unrotated) (Faktoı Extraction: Principal components (Marked loadings are >,700000)		
	Factor 1	Factor 2	Factor 3
X1	-0,734386	0,478628	0,335909
X2	-0,813155	0,219968	0,409879
X3	-0,667733	0,510046	0,189359
X4	-0,853791	0,312090	0,198990
X5	-0,803794	-0,239129	-0,416641
X6	-0,719255	-0,412846	-0,403666
X7	-0,741194	-0,170314	-0,570012
X8	-0,148481	-0,766698	0,443965
X9	-0,274842	-0,887968	0,106588
X10	-0,192353	-0,853229	0,396084
Expl.Var	4,222737	2,995961	1,383086
Prp.Totl	0,422274	0,299596	0,138309

In the lowest row we see a part of variance explained by each factor (**Prp.Totl.**). Thus, the percent of explained variance equals to **Prp.Totl*100**. Close the window.

7. Return to the *Factor Analysis: Resylts* window. Press the *Loading* tag. In the *Factor rotation* field choose the *Varimax normalized* rotation. Initiate the *Plot of Loadings 3D* button again, the plot of loadings 3D where three significant factors with a certain set of variables are highlighted will be displayed on the screen:

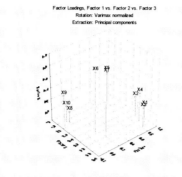

8. Close the plot. Press the *Summary: Factor loading* button. In the table the correlations of variables and highlighted factors are displayed.

Variable	Factor Loadings (Varimax normalized) (Faktor) Extraction: Principal components (Marked loadings are >,700000)		
	Factor 1	Factor 2	Factor 3
X1	0,927031	-0,111483	0,097097
X2	0,907626	0,158708	0,169216
X3	0,818488	-0,222841	0,149295
X4	0,874086	-0,017699	0,318773
X5	0,286181	0,134477	0,681404
X6	0,152435	0,273800	0,867476
X7	0,193883	-0,011335	0,930360
X8	-0,009277	0,898271	-0,000486
X9	-0,136504	0,854797	0,355070
X10	-0,038780	0,955457	0,086487
Expl.Var	3,280071	2,631234	2,690480
Prp.Totl	0,328007	0,263123	0,269048

Now we can interpret the obtained solution. If factor loadings are greater than 0.75, it corresponds with the strong correlation between parameters and factors. The obtained results show that the health level of patients is defined with the help of three factors with a certain set of variables. *Factor* 1 includes the variables X2, X3, X4. *Factor* 2 includes the variables X8, X9, X10. *Factor* 3 includes the variables X5, X6, X7. All factors are defined consequently. As the total variance of *Factor* 1 is larger than the one of the other factors, *Factor* 1 is more correlated with variables rather than *Factors* 2 *and* 3. Close the table.

When the number of factors and variables included in these factors is chosen correctly, the factor loadings tables unite the variables into groups for which correlation coefficients with factors take on the higher values in one group and the lower ones in the other group. For example, the variables X1, X2, X3, X4 have the greatest loadings with Factor 1, but the smaller loadings with Factors 2 and 3, etc. Use other characteristics of factor analysis. Close the table.

9. Go back to the *Factor Analysis:Resylts* window and choose the *Explained variance* tag. Press the *Eigenvalues* button.

170

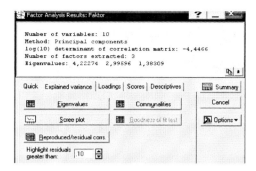

The table of eigenvalues will be displayed. Analyze them taking into account the percent of total variance, i.e. evaluate them according the first and the second criteria.

	Extraction: Principal components			
Value	Eigenvalue	% Total variance	Cumulative Eigenvalue	Cumulative %
1	4,222737	42,22737	4,222737	42,22737
2	2,995961	29,95961	7,218698	72,18698
3	1,383086	13,83086	8,601785	86,01785

In the first column of the table there are eigenvalues, in the second one there is the percent of total variance corresponding to these eigenvalues, then, there are cumulative or accumulated eigenvalues (eigenvalues are summarized 4.22 + 2.99 = 7.21, etc.). Eigenvalues are displayed in decreasing order which reflects the degree of significance of the corresponding highlighted factors to explain the variance of initial data. So, *Factor* 1 that maximum eigenvalue equals to 4.2227 describes approximately 29.95% of the total variance, etc.

According to the Kaiser criterion all three factors can be included in the model, as their eigenvalues are greater than 1, ant the total variance explained by all factors is larger than 86%. To use the Cattell criterion (*Scree-test*), draw the linear plot of dependence between eigenvalues and their number. The point coordinates in which the decrease of dependence decelerates in a stronger way defines the number of factors. Close the table.

10.   Return to the *Factor Analysis:Resylts* window, and choose the *Explained variance* tag. Press the *Scree plot* button.

The scree plot that demonstrates the reasons for excluding all three factors will be displayed. On the *X*-axis there are eigenvalues' numbers, and on the *Y*-axis there are corresponding to them eigenvalues.

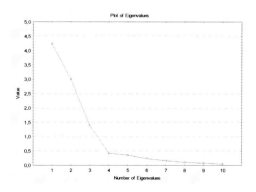

According to the Cattell criterion, it is reasonable to extract such number of factors after which this plot becomes smooth, and eigenvalues become smaller than 1. Here, the *Number of*

171

Eigenvalues point has the value 3 that proves that the extraction of just 3 factors is correct. The fourth point has the value 0.5. Close the analysis window.

7.3.3. METHOD OF PRINCIPLE FACTORS

While the method of principle components is aimed at explaining the total multidimensional variability of the variables by the first m components, the method of principle factors is pointed at explaining the pair connectivity and co-variability between the variables by the first m factors, i.e. recreating the correlation, though the correlation between the extraneous factors is not conformal.

Continuation of the example 7.2

1.   In the menu choose ***Multivariate exploratory techniques –Factor analysis***.

2.   Then, in the ***Factor Analysis*** window in the ***Input file*** field set ***Raw Data***. Switch on ***MD deletion – Casewise.*** Press the ***Variables*** button. Set the variables from 1 to 10 with the help of the ***Select All*** button. Press **OK**.

In the ***Define Method of Factor Extraction*** window press the ***Advanced*** button. Set the maximum number of factors that equals to 3. The ***Mini. Eigenvalue*** field defines the limit which serves the starting point when the eigenvalues will be excluded from the further analysis. Leave the value 1. In the ***Principal factor analysis*** group of options the following ways of evaluation of factor loadings are offered:

- ***Communalities=multiple R?*** is the square of multiple correlation coefficient, and it is a part of explained variance for the corresponding variables in the set number of factors;
- ***Iterated communalities (MINRES)*** or relative variance of minimum residuals;
- ***Maximum likelihood factors;***
- ***Centroid method;***
- ***Principal axis method.***

3.   Choose ***Centroid method.*** In the ***Min. change in communality*** field leave the value 0.01 accessible for both ***Principal axis method*** and ***Centroid method.*** Aiming at the search of maximum possible number of iterations, set 50. The widow will take on the following form:

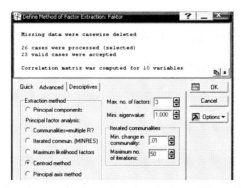

4.   Press **OK**. The ***Factor Analysis:Resylts*** window will be displayed.

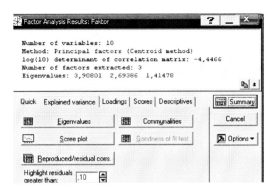

Analyze the results similarly to the previous example, choosing one-by-one necessary tags and buttons.

5.　　Choose the *Loadings* tag. In the *Factor rotation* field leave the factor loadings *Unrotated*, i.e. do not rotate them. Press the *Plot of Loadings 3D* button. The plot shows that the factors are not highlighted. The groups of variables are set on the even basis. Close the window.

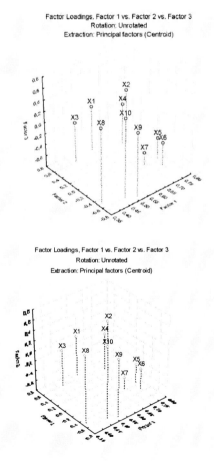

6.　　In the *Factor Analysis:Resylts* window press the *Summary: Factor loading* button. The table of the numerical values of loadings will be displayed. Loadings that are greater than

0.7 are highlighted with red. It is seen that too many variables are not included in any of three factors.

Variable	Factor Loadings (Unrotated) (Faktor) Extraction: Principal factors (Centroid) (Marked loadings are >,700000)		
	Factor 1	Factor 2	Factor 3
X1	0,586737	0,711028	-0,005034
X2	0,745404	0,526873	0,168696
X3	0,475105	0,620996	-0,093056
X4	0,726655	0,543076	-0,070943
X5	0,768351	-0,138552	-0,428745
X6	0,751312	-0,327499	-0,397391
X7	0,687838	-0,153577	-0,579111
X8	0,370331	-0,486729	0,505411
X9	0,516521	-0,691864	0,317258
X10	0,471676	-0,603751	0,582578
Expl.Var	3,908011	2,693858	1,414777
Prp.Totl	0,390801	0,269386	0,141478

It is impossible to interpret the data from neither the plot nor the table.

7.   In the *Factor Analysis:Resylts* window choose the *Loading* tag. In the *Factor rotation* field choose the *Varimax normalized* rotation. The system will rotate the factors using the method of normalized maximum value of variance. Initiate the *Plot of Loadings* 3D button again, and the plot of loadings 3D will be displayed. It is seen that after rotation the variables are grouped into three factors.

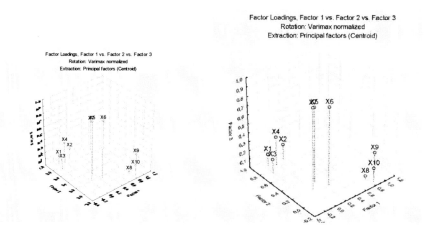

8.   Close the window and return to the *Factor Analysis:Resylts* window. Choose the *Loading* tag and press the *Summary: Factor loading* button. Look at the obtained numerical values of loadings.

Variable	Factor Loadings (Varimax normalized) (l Extraction: Principal factors (Centroid) (Marked loadings are >,700000)		
	Factor 1	Factor 2	Factor 3
X1	-0,138921	0,902487	0,126751
X2	0,157561	0,900038	0,163667
X3	-0,198566	0,746948	0,150535
X4	-0,022405	0,852756	0,316696
X5	0,145610	0,299134	0,826256
X6	0,267172	0,153389	0,857167
X7	0,015264	0,207020	0,888249
X8	0,792147	-0,028425	0,034430
X9	0,850241	-0,126175	0,327557
X10	0,958325	-0,036236	0,081796
Expl.Var	2,445664	3,083581	2,487400
Prp.Totl	0,244566	0,308358	0,248740

In the table, as well as on the plot, three significant factors (with the greatest loadings) with the same set of variables in each factor as in the method of ***Principal components*** are displayed. The part of explained variance (***Prp.Totl)*** is a little bit changed, and the columns of the table are transposed.

9. Close the window and return to the ***Factor Analysis:Resylts*** window. Choose the ***Quick*** tag and the ***Eigenvalues*** button. The analysis table will be displayed.

Value	Eigenvalues (Faktor) Extraction: Principal factors (Centroid)			
	Eigenvalue	% Total variance	Cumulative Eigenvalue	Cumulative %
1	3,908011	39,08011	3,908011	39,08011
2	2,693858	26,93858	6,601869	66,01869
3	1,414777	14,14777	8,016646	80,16646

The table shows that the results of analysis coincide with the results obtained by the principal components method. The ***Factor 1*** has the largest eigenvalue 3.9, and the variance explained by its influence is 39.08%, etc. The total variance explained by all three factors is larger than 80%.

So, after the analysis, look at the factors one more time and decide in what factor this or that variables are included. How do we call the characteristics corresponding to these variables? Judging from the content of characteristics, try to understand for which reason some of them are included in different factors. Give each factor its name. It should summarize all characteristics that are included in the factor or should serve the reason for the correlation between these characteristics. For instance, if the variables $X8$, $X9$, $X10$ in ***Factor*** 2 reflect the testosterone, estrone, and estradiol levels in points, ***Factor*** 2 should be named as *Hormonal*. Perhaps, ***Factor*** 3 will be named as *Anthropo-constitutive*, if it includes the evaluation of such parameters as weight, height, mass, etc. Sometimes the name of one of the characteristics included in the factor may be the name for this factor.

It may happen that the content of the factor does not entirely correspond to the common meaning of the word that has been given as the name of this factor. It is logical because often factors have a complex content that, in this case, depends on the sampling of those things that were understood under these characteristics. If you cannot name the factors with one word, enumerate the components that are included in these factors. For example, if the factor contains 4 characteristics, and it is clear that two of them can be united under the same name (e.g. psychosomatic condition), and two other characteristics can be united under another name, we can conclude that the factor contains two meaningful units. Probably, one of them causes another one. Then, the name of the factor may consist of two words.

7.4. DISCRIMINANT ANALYSIS

Discriminant analysis is an alternative to the multiple regression analysis in such cases when a dependent variable is a non-quantitative (nominative) variable. Here, discriminant analysis solves the same problems as the multiple regression analysis, namely it predicts the values of the dependent variable and defines which independent variables suit better for this prediction. At the same time, discriminant analysis can be defined as a method of classification, as the dependent variable is nominative, i.e. it classifies test subjects into groups corresponding to its various gradations.

The objective of discriminant analysis is to relate some object to one of the classes that have been built earlier, and also to check the consistency of the classification. That is why this analysis is also called the analysis containing learning samples for distinguishing the classifications with teaching. But the term 'discrimination' means not only the divisions of objects into classes, but also the limitation of such division.

Cluster analysis has a disadvantage, namely the absence of the rules and certain criteria to evaluate the quality of classification. At the same time, both the rules and criteria are especially important in diagnostics of rare unusual pathologic processes which have rather unclear symptoms, or in the process of emergency medical response, when a doctor needs to diagnose a patient very quickly. Discriminant analysis helps to solve these problems.

Discriminant analysis consists of several stages.

The first stage is to form the teaching data. The objects with some certain symptoms and accurately made diagnosis (hypertension I, hypertension II, etc.) are gathered. Diagnosis is not a nominative variable. The number of features for classification is not limited, but in the computer programs a limited number of the most informative features are selected automatically. The features that are included in the observation matrix can be both qualitative and quantitative. However, to analyze them it is necessary to convert qualitative features into interval scale according to the degree of their manifestation. The fidelity of information will determine the accuracy of the determinative rules of diagnostics, i.e. the accuracy of classification.

At the second stage statistics package works out the determinative rules of diagnostics in the form of the set of linear classification functions (LCF) and canonical linear discriminant functions (CLDF), and also it evaluates their informational content. A patient relates to the certain class according to the set of symptoms with the help of estimated functions. To visualize estimation, the plot reflecting the order of objects belonging to different classes is displayed in coordinates of the two most significant CLDF.

At the third stage the classification is realized on the basis of the worked out determinative rules. After examination a patient is related to this or that group of diseases.

Let us emphasize the objectives of discriminant analysis one more time:

1. To classify objects. The goal of classification is to determine the significance of discriminant functions and obtain such linear combination of discriminant functions that will allow relating each new object to one of the classes with the known probability on the basis of the data about the known objects.

2. To interpret the differences between classes, i.e. to answer the following questions: how much does this set of variables help to differentiate one class from the other? Which of these variables are more important for differentiating the classes?

Discriminant analysis may be based on both parametric and non-parametric criteria. In parametric methods when the distribution of features is normal in each set, this procedure is based on the mean values in samples. Non-parametric methods of discriminant analysis are based on the ranks, and it is not required to know about the normality of distribution.

Linear discriminative analysis can be presented on the plot as following:

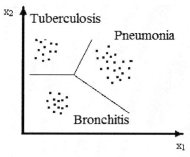

Fig.7.3

However, linear discriminative analysis does not work, for example, in such cases as:

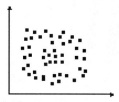

Fig.7.4

Algorithm of parametric discriminant analysis
     1.   To check whether the sampling is created in the interval scales or in the ratio scales, and to understand whether the distribution of features is normal or not.
     2.   To check whether the sampling is divided into finite number (not less than two) of non-intersecting classes, and to point out whether the probability of belonging to this or that class for each object is known.
     3.   To check the absence of correlation between the variables with the help of correlation matrix. If there is dependence between the mean variances or standard deviations (multicollinearity), there is no single-value measure of the relative significance of variables.
     4.   In each class there must be at least two objects from the learning sampling, and the number of discriminant variables must not exceed the value of learning sampling except for two objects.
     Note. *Moderate deviations from the features of normality and correlation are acceptable. After checking the conditions, we can proceed to discrimination. Let us consider the main methods of discriminant analysis realized in the majority of statistics packages:*
- Fisher Linear discriminant analysis (LDA);
- Canonical discriminant analysis;
- Distance Analysis;
- Stepwise Discriminant Analysis.

Fisher Linear discriminant analysis
     This method was introduced by R.Fisher, and, here, the related functions are called Fisher's linear classification functions (LCF). The k linear functions are built, and the object relates to k-class, if the value of k function is maximum on it. Classification functions should not be mixed up with canonical linear discriminant functions (CLDF). Classification functions serves to define which group each object is more likely to be related to. The number of classifications equals to the number of groups. The values of linear classification functions are estimated for each object and each population by the formula:

$$d_{mk} = a_k + b_{k1}x_{1k} + b_2 x_{2k} + \dots + b_n x_{nk} \quad or \quad d_{mk} = a_k + \sum b_{ki} \cdot x_{mi} \quad m = 1,\dots n; \quad k = 1,\dots g,$$

where k denotes the corresponding group, m denotes the number of the object, coefficients b_{ki} are called the scales for i-variable when estimating the classification value for k population; d_{mk} is the value of LGF for m-object in the group k, a_k is an absolute term of an equation; x_{mi} is the observed value of i-variable for the corresponding m-object in the group k. The observation is ascribed to that group for which classification function has the maximum value.

Canonical discriminant analysis or probability method relates the object to class k, if the corresponding posteriori probability of this relation is maximum. Linear discriminant functions applied in these methods are often called canonical (CLDF). This analysis has the algorithm which is opposite to the first type of analysis. Here, the distribution of the objects is realized according to the minimum values of discriminant function. The object relates to the certain class only if the *Euclidean distances* from the center of cluster to the evaluated parameter are minimum. This type of analysis is, of course, more complicated and time-consuming.

Linear discriminant function is written as:

$$D_{mk}=a_k+ b_1x_1+b_2x_2+... + b_nx_n , \quad m=1,....n; \quad k=1,....g$$

It is called canonical linear discriminant function with the unknown coefficients b_{ki}. where D_{km} is the value of the canonical discriminant function for m-object in the group k; a_k is the absolute term of the equation; x_{mi} is the observed value of i-variable for the corresponding m-object in the group k. The constants b_{ki} are coefficients that we are to evaluate with the help of discriminant analysis. In statistics packages these functions are denoted as **Root**. The goal of discriminant analysis is to determine such unknown coefficients that will allow us to divide into groups very accurately, knowing the values of discriminant function. Coefficients of the first canonical discriminant function are chosen in such a way that centroids of different groups must differ from each other as much as possible. Coefficients of the second group are chosen the same way, but here one more condition is added, namely there must not be any correlation between the values of the second and the first functions. The other functions are determined the same way. If the number of predictors is enough, the number of function will be one unit smaller than the number of groups. While searching each following function, the absence of correlation between it and all previous functions is required. If the number of groups equals to G, the number of canonical discriminant functions will be one unit smaller than the number of groups (G - 1). However, there are many reasons of practical character that make it useful to have one, two or even three functions. In this case graphic presentation of the objects will be presented in 1D, 2D or 3D spaces. In the particular case, when k = 2, the hypersurface is a line, and when k = 3, it is a plane. If, for example, we consider the case with three classes, the values of discriminant function are laid off in the plane, namely **Root 1** is laid on the one axis, and **Root 2** is laid on the other axis.

When the evaluation of statistical significance of each canonical function has been made, and it has been determined which functions play the most significant role in discrimination, the values of these functions for each observed object are estimated. The smallest value is applied in classification. It is compared with the mean values of distances to centroids of each group. The object belongs to the group the distance to which coincides with the estimated value of CLDF.

When we apply the maximum likelihood method on default, two sets of evaluation are used for optimal classification, namely:
- **Posteriori probabilities of belonging to a class** that can be considered as the main rule applied when there is no additional information about the objects.
- **Conditional probabilities of belonging to a class** where each of them equals to the probability of obtaining the corresponding value of discriminant function when the object belongs to the class. The assumption that the values of discriminant functions are distributed normally is used.

$P(G_i)$ is the posteriori probability of belonging of the observation to the group G_i which is the estimation of probability when some information about the objects of class G_i is absent. Posteriori probability can be estimated by different methods. In case of representative sampling as the estimation of posteriori probabilities, the parts of objects in each class can be used. For example, if the sample volume is 1000 observation where 600 (60%) observation belong to the class 1, and 400 (40%) belongs to the class 2, the posteriori probability of class 1 equals to 0.6, and the one of class 2 equals to 0.4.

If the researcher does not have any information about probability at all, and the chance to belong to all groups is the same, then posteriori probabilities may be treated as equal to each other. Each observation must belong to some group that is why the sum of posteriori probabilities equals to 1. In case of two classes, posteriori probabilities will equal to 0.5, and in case of five classes, they will be 0.2.

Posteriori probabilities contain some information about the probability of belonging to the certain group, but they do not take into account the peculiarities of each separate observation. To take them into account, it is necessary to estimate probabilities considering the additional data about the observation. If, for example, the values of discriminant function have normal distribution in each class, first of all, we assume that the observations belong to the group G_1, and estimate the probability of the fact that the discriminant function takes on the value D. Then, we suggest that the observations belong to the group G_2, and repeat the estimations. Each of these probabilities will be called the conditional probability of the value D for this class, and it will be denoted as $P(D/G_i)$. The conditional probability of the value D for this class shows how much it is possible for the members of the class to obtain this value exactly.

Probability of belonging of observation to each class under observation is estimated with the help of posteriori probability $P(G_i/D)$ according to the **Bayes**' theorem using the probabilities $P(D/G_i)$ and $P(G_i)$. Posteriori probability assigns the optimal rule of classification, namely the observation should be related to the class for which the posteriori probability D is maximum.

$$P(G_i / D) = \frac{P(D/G_i)P(G_i)}{\sum_{i=1}^{g} P(D/G_i)P(G_i)}$$

Distance analysis considerss the objects as the points in *Euclidean distances*. The smaller the distance between objects is, the greater the similarity is. However, when the variables are correlated, measured in different units, and have different standard deviations, it is hard to define the notion of 'distance'. In this case, it is useful to apply *Mahalanobis distances* instead of Euclidean *distances*.

The observed analyses suppose the simultaneous insert of all variables. In this case each independent variable is taken into account, while its discriminant power is not. Stepwise discriminant analysis is the alternative to it when the variables are inserted consequently, considering their ability to discriminate groups. When stepwise analysis supposes 'inclusions', in every step we look through all variables, and find the one that contributes much to the discrimination of populations. This variable must be included in the model at the given stage, and then, we proceed to the next stage.

In stepwise analysis with 'exclusion' we move vice versa. In this case all variables, firstly, will be included in the model, and, then, in every step the variables that do not play a significant role in differentiating will be excluded. So, if the analysis is successful, only important variables will be saved in the model, i.e. those variables that play the most significant role in discrimination. Stepwise discriminant analysis is based on the use of the significance level of F-statistics. It is simple enough in its realization when the data is processed on the computer, and it helps us to estimate the quality of the obtained classification, as it is also an additional method to two methods mentioned above.

To form informational database of discriminant analysis it is necessary to solve two problems mentioned above with the help of the following steps:
- To estimate the quality of built classification and decide how much it is sensitive to the division of objects into classes, and how much this discrimination is reliable.
- To build classification matrix with evaluation of sensitivity of the groups towards the teaching data.
- To evaluate the informativeness of symptoms included and not included in the linear classification functions.

- To find out which of them have the highest value for correct qualitative discrimination.
  - To identify the coefficients of linear classification functions (LCF).
  - To identify the contribution of CLDF to the variance of symptoms.
  - To find the coefficients of CLDF
  - To identify the factor structure of CLDF.
  - To find out the coordinates of the centroids of the groups.
  - To draw the plot of the placement of the objects under analysis.

After completing these steps, the procedure of the diagnostics of some certain patients consists of the estimation of either LCF or CLDF to relate a certain patient to this or that group of deceases.

Example 7.3. Hypotheriosis treatment outcome

22 people who suffered from hypotheriosis were divided into three groups:
- **Group 1.** Treatment is not successful, i.e. patient's condition remains the same.
- **Group 2.** Treatment is successful. Clinical examination shows that patient has been cured.
- **Group 3.** Treatment outcome is successful, but relapse may happen in the future.

From the results of observation we know the belonging of patients to the groups (classes), and also there are the following measurements (table 7-4):
- x_1 – iodine that is found in 3 hours after taking the test dose;
- x_2 – iodine that is found in 48 hours after taking the test dose;
- x_3 – protein-bound iodine level in blood in 48 hours.

Table 7-4

Protein-bound iodine level in blood plasma of the patients with hypotheriosis

x_1	x_2	x_3	Group
55.8	48	2.74	1
75	60	1.37	1
72	65	0.7	1
65	58.7	2.1	1
70	63	1,5	1
52.7	50	0.53	2
20.8	22.3	0.13	2
14	3.1	0.18	2
27	41.7	0.19	2
44.3	63.8	0.22	2
47.5	50.1	0.29	2
54	57	0.19	2
16.1	20.6	0.22	2
57.5	74.5	0.49	2
55.8	55	0.74	2
46.5	66	0.22	2
43.2	55	0.01	2
14.4	40.1	0.18	3
20.1	32.1	0.17	3
24.1	16.9	0.12	3
16.3	32.1	0.36	3
20.5	34.4	0.35	3

180

Work order

1.   Launch the Statistica program. Input the data from the table 7-4.

2.   In the menu choose ***Statistics–Multivariate Exploratory Techniques– Discriminant Analysis.***

3.   In the ***Discriminant Function Analysis*** window press the ***Variables*** button. Choose the ***Grouping variable*** – group and the ***Independent variable list – X1-X8***. Press **OK**.

4.   In the ***Discriminant Function Analysis*** window set the ***Advanced options*** option and also ***MD deletion – Casewise.*** Press the ***Codes for grouping variable*** button. In the displayed window press the buttons **ALL** and **OK**. As the results of all manipulations, the final window will look like as following:

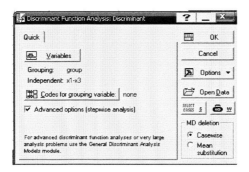

5.   Press **OK**. The ***Model Definition*** window will be displayed. Choose the ***Advanced*** tag. In the ***Method*** field choose ***Forward stepwise***. The rest parameters are set on default (do not change these parameters). Press **OK**.

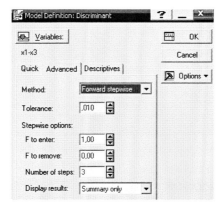

6.   In the new ***Discriminant Function Analysis Results*** window in the header the criterion $F = 10.59$ and $p<0.0000$ is inserted. It proves the statistical significance of the model.

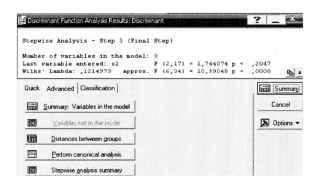

7.   Analyze the structure of the correlation between groups. Choose the *Advanced* tag and press the *Distances between groups* button. The window of analysis with three tables will be displayed. According to the *Squared Mahalanobis distances* table data, we can judge about the quality of the model classification. The larger the distance, the more qualitative the discrimination of observation and the degree of differences of the groups are. It is seen from the table that the centers of the groups are consequently placed in 3D space corresponding to the group number. The distances between groups increase consequently.

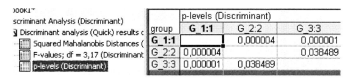

Choose the *p-levels* table and analyze the statistical dependence of such variables as *Mahalanobis distances*. *P-levels* are lower than critical 0.05 for all values of distances.

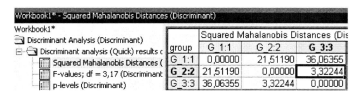

8.   Close the table. Choose the *Quick* tag. Press the *Variables in the model* button. The table highlights two most informative variables (symptoms). They are the variables x_1 and x_3. In the first column there are the values of the Λ-*Wilks's* coefficient for the whole model appeared after the exclusion of the variable. The larger the value, the more desirable this variable in the discrimination procedure. Thus, the variables are desirable in the following order: x_3, x_1, x_2. In the second column there are the values of Λ- *Wilks's* that equals to the correlation between 'Λ- *Wilks's* after the addition of the variable' and 'Λ- *Wilks's* before the addition of the variable'. Λ-*Wilks's* characterizes a single contribution of the corresponding variable in the separation power of the model. The smaller the value is, the greater the contribution of this variable to the total discrimination is. Thus, the variables are placed in the following order according to the power of discrimination: x_3, x_1, x_2. *F-remove* is the value of the Fisher's criterion with the corresponding levels of significance. The lower *F-remove* and higher *p-levels* are, the less desirable the variables in the model are. The variables with $p>0.05$ may be excluded from the model. This is the variable x_2.

	Discriminant Function Analysis Summary (Discriminant) Step 3, N of vars in model: 3; Grouping: group (3 grps) Wilks' Lambda: ,12150 approx. F (6,34)=10,590 p< ,0000					
N=22	**Wilks'** Lambda	Partial Lambda	F-remove (2,17)	p-level	Toler.	1-Toler. (R-Sqr.)
x3	0,246376	0,493138	8,736547	0,002456	0,999678	0,000322
x1	0,225000	0,539989	7,241068	0,005312	0,304640	0,695360
x2	0,146427	0,829748	1,744074	0,204665	0,304666	0,695334

9.   Estimate the informativiness of the variables that are not included in the model. To do this, close the window of analysis. Press the *Advanced* button and the *Variables not in the model* button. In our example there are no such variables, that is why this button is not active.

10.   In the *Discriminant Function Analysis Results* window choose the *Classification* tag and press the *Classification functions* button.

The table *Classification functions* in which each symptom corresponds to the set of coefficients for linear classification function (LCF) will be displayed.

Variable	Classification Functions; grouping: group (Disc		
	G_1:1 p=,22727	G_2:2 p=,54545	G_3:3 p=,22727
x3	11,3069	2,01399	1,62343
x1	0,6113	0,20975	-0,01228
x2	-0,1753	0,03237	0,11835
Constant	-26,4738	-5,83621	-3,39753

For example, the coefficient 11.3069 will stand before the variable x_3 in the first equation, and in the second equation the variable x_3 must be multiplied by the coefficient 2.01399, etc. In the bottom line there are the values of the absolute term of the equation for each classification function (*Constant*). Using this table, we can calculate linear classification functions (LCF) by the following formulas:

$$d_1 = -26.4738 + 11.3069 \times x_3 + 0.6113 \times x_1 - 0.1753 \times x_2$$
$$d_2 = -5.83621 + 2.01399 \times x_3 + 0.20975 \times x_1 + 0.03237 \times x_2$$
$$d_3 = -3.39753 + 1.62343 \times x_3 - 0.01228 \times x_1 + 0.11835 \times x_2$$

Having substituted the values of the symptoms codes of a certain patient into equation, we can calculate linear classification function (LCF), and, then, we can relate the disease to the certain class according to its maximum value.

11.   Close the table. In the *Discriminant Function Analysis Results* window press the *Classification* tag and the *Classification matrix* button. The table containing the information about the sensitivity of the main rules of discriminations will be displayed.

Group	Classification Matrix (Discriminant) Rows: Observed classifications Columns: Predicted classifications			
	Percent Correct	G_1:1 p=,22727	G_2:2 p=,54545	G_3:3 p=,22727
G_1:1	100,0000	5	0	0
G_2:2	91,6667	0	11	1
G_3:3	80,0000	0	1	4
Total	90,9091	5	12	5

The matrix rows are the initial classes of patients, and the columns are the predicted classes of patients. The percent of correct classification of objects is an additional measure of differences between groups, and it can be treated as the most suitable measure of discrimination.

Notice that the value of percentage is applicable to estimate the correct prediction only if the distribution of the objects into groups has been random. For instance, if the classification is random, 50% can be predicted for two groups, and 25% can be predicted for four groups. Thus, if the *Total is* 60% of the correct prediction for two groups, this value must be treated as too small, while it shows good separation ability in case of four groups. It is seen from the table that the accuracy of diagnostics by the main rules (the total percent of the correct classification) is 90.9%. 5 objects out of 5 are related to the group G_1, and the percent of total classification is 100%. 11 objects are correctly related to the group G_2 that is 91.67% of the correct classification, and the object 1 is related to the group G_3. 4 objects are correctly related to the group G_3 that is 80% of the correct classification, and one object is related to G_2. The data speaks of good separation ability of this model. Diagnostics of the second and the third groups is not accurate enough as the overlap of the symptoms engenders the need in much more accurate discrimination of this decease. Close the table.

To find out the nature of discrimination it is necessary to make canonical analysis, i.e. to find canonical linear classification functions *(Root).*

10. In the *Discriminant Function Analysis Results* window choose the *Advanced* tag. Press the *Perform canonical analysis* button. Choose the *Advanced* tag, and press the *Summary: Chi square tests of successive roots* button.

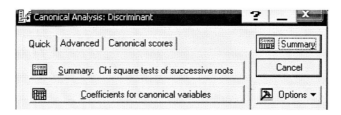

Roots Removed	Chi-Square Tests with Successive Roots Removed (Discriminant)					
	Eigen-value	Canonicl R	Wilks' Lambda	Chi-Sqr.	df	p-level
0	5,444488	0,919146	0,121497	37,94155	6	0,000001
1	0,277159	0,465846	0,782988	4,40349	2	0,110610

The table reflects the contribution of CLDF to the variance of features. To evaluate effectiveness of the canonical discriminant function, the canonical R, Λ- *Wilks's,* χ^2 statistics, and *p-level* are used. The values of discriminant function must separate the groups as clearly as possible. The successfulness of this separation is shown by the correlation coefficient between the estimated values of discriminant function and the index of belonging to the group the square of which shows which part of variance of dependent variable is explained by the model (the same as R^2 in regression analysis).

The first CLDF *(Root)* must describe the greater part of the variance of disease symptoms. The second CLDF describes the greater part of remained features in decreasing order. As it has been already mentioned, the checking of the quality of discrimination is based on the comparison of the average values of discriminant functions for the observed groups. These mean values play a very significant role in discriminant analysis, and they are called centroids. The number of centroids corresponds to the number of groups, i.e. one centroid corresponds to one group. Besides, the values of discriminant function are called *discriminant scores. Before interpreting discriminant function, we need to check its statistical significance. To do this, the null hypothesis about the equality of centroids in all groups is checked (this hypothesis must be rejected for this discriminant function to be statistically significant). This hypothesis is checked with the help of Wilks' lambda. This coefficient takes on the values from 0 to 1, and the closer to zero it is, the better the results of discrimination are. Thus, Λ- Wilks's* helps us to test whether the difference between the mean values of discriminant function is significant or not.

To estimate the significance of the difference, the eigenvalues of discriminant function are used, and they are shown under the name **Eigenvalue.** It corresponds to the relation of the sum of the square of the variance between the groups to the sum of the square of the variance inside the groups. If the eigenvalue is large, it proves the high quality of the function. The first CLDF has the larger eigenvalue. The power of contribution of function is evaluated with the help of χ^2. In the mentioned example the value $p < 0.05$ indicates that the power is statistically significant.

Conclusion: to solve the problems of medical diagnostics, two CLDF (with the level of significance **p**<0.05) should be applied. Close the window of analysis.

12.   In the *Canonical Analysis* window choose the *Advanced* tag and press the *Coefficients for canonical variables* button. The *CLDF* table will be displayed.

Variable	Raw Coefficients (Discriminant) for Canonical Variables	
	Root 1	**Root 2**
x3	-1,77581	1,758029
x1	-0,09772	-0,073116
x2	0,04759	0,016846
Constant	2,91958	1,221231
Eigenval	5,44449	0,277159
Cum.Prop	0,95156	1,000000

Two tables are displayed, namely *Raw Coefficients* and *Standardized Coefficients*. We are going to use just the first table *Raw Coefficients* for the further analysis. To solve the problems of the medical diagnostics, in this example the two first CLDF (**Root 1** and **Root 2**) should be applied with the cumulative contribution into variance of the symptoms equaling to 95.156% and 100% as it is seen from the table. The function 1 is more significant as it is responsible for 95.156% of the explained variance. The function 2 is responsible for 4.84% of the explained variance (100% - 95.156%). Constant is the absolute term of the equation in every CLDF.

The coefficients should be placed into two CLDF.

$D_1 = 2.91958 - 1.77581 \times x_3 - 0.09772 \times x_1 + 0.04759 \times x_2$
$D_2 = 1.221231 + 1.758029 \times x_3 - 0.073116 \times x_1 + 0.016846 \times x_2$

Having placed the values of the symptom codes of the certain patient, it is possible to calculate CLDF. The patient for whose D_1 and D_2 are defined according to his/her symptoms should be related to the group by the minimum distance from the corresponding centroid (look at the table of centroids). Close the window.

13.   In the *Canonical Analysis* window choose the *Advanced* tag and press the *Factor structure* button. The table with the coefficients of factor structure called *Factor Structure Matrix* will be displayed.

Variable	Factor Structure Matrix (Discriminant) Correlations Variables - Canonical Roots (Pooled-within-groups correlations)	
	Root 1	Root 2
x3	-0,682284	0,697920
x1	-0,570115	-0,711299
x2	-0,231237	-0,507064

Factor Structure Matrix allows us to find out which variables mark or define a separate discriminant function. The coefficients of *Factor Structure Matrix* are the correlations between the variables in the model and the discriminant function. They can be perceived as the factor loadings of the variables for each discriminant function. Usually structure coefficients are used for substantial interpretation of discriminant functions, while coefficients of discriminant functions denote the contribution of each variable to the function. The variables x_1 and x_3 have moderate correlation with *Root* 1 and *Root* 2. Close the table.

15. Find out the coordinates of centroids for four groups. In the *Canonical Analysis* window choose the *Advanced* tag and press the *Means of canonical variable* button.

Group	Means of Canonical Variables (Discriminar	
	Root 1	Root 2
G_1:1	-3,86459	0,231411
G_2:2	0,72819	-0,415303
G_3:3	2,11692	0,765317

The obtained table contains means of canonical variables, i.e. the coordinates of centroids of the corresponding groups.

16. In the *Canonical Analysis* window choose the *Canonical scores* tag and press the *Scatterplot of canonical scores* button.

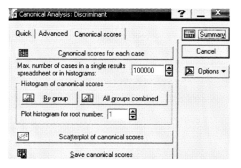

17. In the displayed *Select canonical roots for* window in the *First root* field set (if it is not set on default) *Root* 1. In the *Second root* field set *Root* 2. Press **Ok**.

The plot of the placement of the four groups will be displayed in the coordinates of the first and the second canonical CLDF.

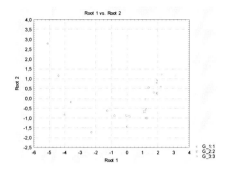

In this example *Root* **1** mostly discriminates between the classes 1 and 2, to be more accurate, between the class 1 and the union of the classes 2 and 3. The classes 2 and 3 are discriminated with each other in not so obvious manner. In the *y*-axis (*Root* **2**) we see the shift of the points of the classes 2 and 3 relatively to the central line (0). The patient for whom D_1 and D_2 (*Root* **1** and *Root* **2**) are defined by his/her symptoms should be related to the group by the minimum distance from the corresponding centroid. Close the table. Close the *Canonical Analysis* window.

18. In the package **Statistica** not only a graphical way of defining the distances to centroids is possible, but also there is a way of estimation of so-called *Mahalanobis distances*. Return to the *Discriminant Function Analysis Results* window, choose the *Classification* tag, and press the *Squared Mahalanobis distance* button.

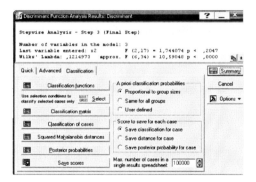

The table (*Squared Mahalanobis distance*) with the squares of *Mahalanobis distance* from the points (cases) to the center of the groups will be displayed.

Case	Observed Classif.	Squared Mahalanobis Distances from Group Incorrect classifications are marked with *		
		G_1:1 p=,22727	G_2:2 p=,54545	G_3:3 p=,22727
1	G_1:1	8,16590	44,44129	56,47834
2	G_1:1	1,54748	22,79523	40,22477
3	G_1:1	6,44990	10,75922	25,47342
4	G_1:1	1,25882	28,58337	42,36599
5	G_1:1	0,27328	18,67574	33,47062
6	G_2:2	10,82888	2,70953	11,29978
7	G_2:2	32,21204	2,54552	1,42075
8	G_2:2	33,05452	6,83113	6,02731
9	G_2:2	33,72718	2,09706	0,43641
10	G_2:2	28,29380	1,93518	4,18010
11	G_2:2	17,41043	0,61298	6,68940
12	G_2:2	17,84748	1,54552	9,24378
* 13	G_2:2	34,57792	3,51577	0,66650
14	G_2:2	18,24335	3,05923	9,53681
15	G_2:2	7,69052	3,88696	13,15807
16	G_2:2	27,52564	2,02002	4,86358
17	G_2:2	28,31437	0,82446	3,93009
18	G_3:3	50,72493	9,45476	2,46617
19	G_3:3	36,68000	3,12432	0,03476
* 20	G_3:3	28,45035	3,49103	4,75243
21	G_3:3	38,03905	4,96297	0,33437
22	G_3:3	34,14467	3,30034	0,13351

The case is related to the group the *Mahalanobis distance* to which is minimum.

For example, the case 1 relates to the first class because *Mahalanobis distance* is minimum and it equals to 8.165. Close the window of analysis. While using this main rule, incorrect classified cases are highlighted by the sign *. They are the cases 13 and 20. Note that posteriori probabilities have been set proportionally to the number of groups, and they are 22.7%, 54.5%, 22.7% (look at the column names).

19. Before analysis we set the probability for each group with which it belongs to the certain class. With the completed analysis it is possible to recalculate these probabilities and obtain *the posteriori probability* of classification. In the window *Discriminant Function Analysis Results*.choose the tag *Classification* and press the button *Posterior probabilities*.

The table with posteriori probabilities of belonging of the object to the certain class will be displayed.

Case	Observed Classif.	Posterior Probabilities (Discriminant) Incorrect classifications are marked with *		
		G_1:1 p=,22727	G_2:2 p=,54545	G_3:3 p=,22727
1	G_1:1	1,000000	0,000000	0,000000
2	G_1:1	0,999942	0,000058	0,000000
3	G_1:1	0,782267	0,217675	0,000058
4	G_1:1	0,999997	0,000003	0,000000
5	G_1:1	0,999758	0,000242	0,000000
6	G_2:2	0,007098	0,987293	0,005609
7	G_2:2	0,000000	0,577637	0,422363
8	G_2:2	0,000001	0,616226	0,383773
9	G_2:2	0,000000	0,511284	0,488716
10	G_2:2	0,000092	0,880579	0,119421
11	G_2:2	0,000119	0,991086	0,008795
12	G_2:2	0,000000	0,366058	0,633942
* 13	G_2:2	0,000207	0,983721	0,016072
14	G_2:2	0,058344	0,937865	0,003791
15	G_2:2	0,000001	0,908648	0,091351
16	G_2:2	0,000000	0,918958	0,081041
17	G_3:3	0,000000	0,067937	0,932063
18	G_3:3	0,000000	0,338651	0,661349
19	G_3:3	0,000001	0,818492	0,181507
* 20	G_3:3	0,000000	0,191726	0,808274
21	G_3:3	0,000000	0,330053	0,669947

Table interpretation: in the first column there are the clusters numbers for each case (diagnosis); in the second column there are *posteriori probabilities* of relation of each patient to the certain type of diagnosis. The patient relates to some groups with maximum *posteriori probability*.

For the second patient the first diagnosis (class) is more probable, because it corresponds to the probability equaling to 99.99%.

Example of classification for the certain patient

As a diagnostic example, let us analyze two cases (of two patients) with the symptoms included in the model.

Table 7-5

Diagnostic example

Patients	x_1	x_2	x_3
Patient 1	55.7	49	2.7
Patient 2	23	21	0.15

According to the formulas of CLDF

$D_1 = 2.91958 - 1.77581 \times x_3 - 0.09772 \times x_1 + 0.04759 \times x_2$

$D_2 = 1.221231 + 1.758029 \times x_3 - 0.073116 \times x_1 + 0.016846 \times x_2$

Let us estimate the coordinates for the first patient:

$D_1 = 2.91958 - 1.77581 \times 2.7 - 0.09772 \times 55.7 + 0.04759 \times 49 = -4.99$

$D_2 = 1.221231 + 1.758029 \times 2.7 - 0.073116 \times 55.7 + 0.016846 \times 49 = 2.72$

And for the second one:

$D_1 = 2.91958 - 1.77581 \times 0.15 - 0.09772 \times 23 + 0.04759 \times 21 = 1.4$

$D_2 = 1.221231 + 1.758029 \times 0.15 - 0.073116 \times 23 + 0.016846 \times 21 = 0.16$

If we compare the distance to centroids using the corresponding table, it is understandable that the first patient relates to the class **G 1:1**, and the second patient relates to the class **G 2:2**. The same result may be obtained by placing the points of CLDF for each patient on the plot of centroids.

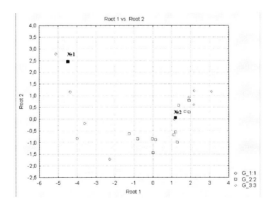

The use of LCF also proves the obtained result. In this case a patient is related to the group for which LCF takes on the maximum value. The estimation of LCF for the first patient shows the following results: $d_1=38,1$; $d_2=11,4$; $d_3=6,1$. d_1 has the maximum value.

The estimation of LCF for the second patient shows the following results: $d_1=-14.4$; $d_2=-0.03$; $d_3=-0.95$. d_2 has the maximum value.

Cross-validation

In the discriminant analysis the main marker is the accuracy of classification, and it can be easily defined by estimating the part of correctly classified observations with the help of prognostic equation.

Cross-validation is a procedure of evaluation of the prognostic accuracy with the help of the data from special testing sampling (the term cross-validation sampling is used as well) by comparing the prognostic accuracy with the one that has been obtained in the sampling according to which the model has been built. So, the model is built with the help of the learning sampling, and the prognostic accuracy is estimated according to the learning sampling on the basis of model. If the researcher deals with quite a big sampling, the following approach is applied: the analysis is done by one part of the data (e.g. by the half of the data), and then, the prognostic equation is applied to classification of observations in the second part of the data. The prognostic accuracy is evaluated by cross-verification. If on the test sampling the model gives the results of the same quality as on the learning sampling, the model is said to succeed in cross-validation. To make cross-validation with the small volume of sampling, the special methods in which testing and learning samplings may be crossed partially have been worked out.

The classification of new cases with the help of the Statistica package

After 22 observations of the data, add two new observations (case 23 and 24) into the table with the initial data and insert the values of their variables from the table 7-5 ignoring the variables that are not included in the model if there are so.

Add Cases			
How many:	2		OK
Insert after case:	22		Cancel
Use 0 to insert before first case.			

22	20,5	34,4	0,35	3
23	55,7	49	2,7	
24	23	21	0,15	

Set the variables again, because they have changed, and also set the stepwise analysis. To understand which class these objects relates to, in the *Discriminant Function Analysis Results* window press the *Posterior probabilities* button again. You will see the table with the posteriori probabilities to which the following rows will be added:

22	G_3:3	0,000000	0,330053	0,669947
23	---	1,000000	0,000000	0,000000
24	---	0,000000	0,715274	0,284726

So, the new observation shows that the first patient can be related to the first class **G 1:1** with 100% probability, and the second one can be related to the class **G 2:2** with 71.52% probability. Close the window.

Press the *Mahalanobis distance* button and you will see the table where two last rows contains the distances of new cases to the group centers:

22	G_3:3	34,14467	3,30034	0,13351
23	---	7,70166	42,73796	54,52740
24	---	29,44895	2,46087	2,55221

190

As the square of the distance from the first patient to the center of classes is minimum for the class **G 1:1**, there is a high possibility that it relates to the first class, and the *Squared Mahalanobis distance* for the second patient is minimum for the class **G 2:2** meaning that it relates to the second class.

If the conditions of classical discriminant analysis are not fulfilled, or the distribution of predicators does not obey the law of normal distribution or they are in the categorical scale, we can use the general discriminant models realized in the **GDA** module of Statistica package.

REFERENCES

1. Banerjee, A. Medical Statistics Made Clear.- Moscow: Practical medicine, 2007. 287 p.
2. Bailey, J. Statistical Methods in Biology.- Moscow: Foreign literature, 1964. 271 p.
3. Bellman, R. E. Mathematical Methods in Medicine.- Moscow: Mir, 1987. 200 p.
4. Borovikov, V.P. STATISTICA. Art computer data analysis: For professionals+ CD. - St. Petersburg:Piter, 2003. 688 p.
5. A. Buhl, P. Zofel, J. SPSS: Information processing. - Moscow: DiaSoft, 2005. 602 p.
6. Glantz, A Biomedical Statistics. - Moscow: Praktika, 1999. 459 p.
7. Glass, G., Stanley, J. Statistical methods in education and psychology. - Moscow: Progress, 1976. 495 p.
8. Greenhalgh, T. The basics of evidence-based medicine. - Moscow: GEOTAR MEDIA, 2006. 240 p.
9. Hollander, M., Wolfe, D.A. Nonparametric statistical methods. - Moscow: Finance and Statistics, 1983. 518 p.
10. Kendall, M.G. Stuart, A. Statistical inference and communication. - Main Edition of Sci. Literature, 1973. 899 p.
11. Petrie, A., Sabin, C. Medical statistics at a glance. - Moscow: GEOTAR-MED, 2003. 141 p.
12. Trukhacheva, N. E-learning in der medizinischen Hochschule und Fragen der Qualität Lehrer/innenbildung in Europa. - Wien, 2008.
13. Trukhacheva, N. E-Learning:Aktueller Stand und Chancen in der medizinischen Bildung in Russland. In:Unterrichtsforschung und Unterrichtsentwicklung. - Zürich: ZU, 2009. S.174-176.
14. Wolff, R., Antes, G.: Evidenzbasierung - Woher kommt die Evidenz und wie wird sie bewertet und genutzt? // Verhaltenstherapie und Psychosoziale Praxis. 2007. № 39. S. 135

Table of Values of The Laplace Function $F(t) = \dfrac{1}{\sqrt{2\pi}} \displaystyle\int_0^t e^{-\frac{t^2}{2}} dt$

t	F(t)	t	F(t)	t	F(t)	t	F(t)
0.00	0.0000	0.32	0.1255	0.64	0.2389	0.96	0.3315
0.01	0.0040	0.33	0.1293	0.65	0.2422	0.97	0.3340
0.02	0.0080	0.34	0.1331	0.66	0.2454	0.98	0.3365
0.03	0.0120	0.35	0.1368	0.67	0.2486	0.99	0.3389
0.04	0.0160	0.36	0.1406	0.68	0.2516	1.00	0.3413
0.05	0.0199	0.37	0.1443	0.69	0.2549	1.01	0.3438
0.06	0.0239	0.38	0.1480	0.70	0.2580	1.02	0.3461
0.07	0.0279	0.39	0.1517	0.71	0.2611	1.03	0.3485
0.08	0.0319	0.40	0.1554	0.72	0.2642	1.04	0.3508
0.09	0.0359	0.41	0.1591	0.73	0.2673	1.05	0.3531
0.10	0.0398	0.42	0.1628	0.74	0.2703	1.06	0.3554
0.11	0.0438	0.43	0.1664	0.75	0.2734	1.07	0.3577
0.12	0.0478	0.44	0.1700	0.76	0.2764	1.08	0.3599
0.13	0.0517	0.45	0.1736	0.77	0.2794	1.09	0.3621
0.14	0.0557	0.46	0.1772	0.78	0.2823	1.10	0.3643
0.15	0.0596	0.47	0.1808	0.79	0.2852	1.11	0.3665
0.16	0.0636	0.48	0.1844	0.80	0.2881	1.12	0.3686
0.17	0.0675	0.49	0.1879	0.81	0.2910	1.13	0.3708
0.18	0.0714	0.50	0.1915	0.82	0.2939	1.14	0.3729
0.19	0.0753	0.51	0.1950	0.83	0.2967	1.15	0.3749
0.20	0.0793	0.52	0.1985	0.84	0.2995	1.16	0.3770
0.21	0.0832	0.53	0.2019	0.85	0.3023	1.17	0.3790
0.22	0.0871	0.54	0.2054	0.86	0.3051	1.18	0.3810
0.23	0.0910	0.55	0.2088	0.87	0.3078	1.19	0.3830
0.24	0.0948	0.56	0.2123	0.88	0.3106	1.20	0.3849
0.25	0.0987	0.57	0.2157	0.89	0.3133	1.21	0.3869
0.26	0.1026	0.58	0.2190	0.90	0.3159	1.22	0.3883
0.27	0.1064	0.59	0.2224	0.91	0.3186	1.23	0.3907
0.28	0.1103	0.60	0.2257	0.92	0.3212	1.24	0.3925
0.29	0.1141	0.61	0.2291	0.93	0.3228	1.25	0.3944
0.30	0.1179	0.62	0.2324	0.94	0.3264	1.26	0.3962
0.31	0.1217	0.63	0.2357	0.95	0.3289	1.27	0.3980

Table of Values Of The Laplace Function F(t) (continuation)

t	F(t)	t	F(t)	t	F(t)	t	F(t)
1.28	0.3997	1.61	0.4463	1.94	0.4738	2.54	0.4945
1.29	0.4015	1.62	0.4474	1.95	0.4744	2.56	0.4948
1.30	0.4032	1.63	0.4484	1.96	0.4750	2.58	0.4951
1.31	0.4049	1.64	0.4495	1.97	0.4756	2.60	0.4953
1.32	0.4066	1.65	0.4505	1.98	0.4761	2.62	0.4956
1.33	0.4082	1.66	0.4515	1.99	0.4767	2.64	0.4959
1.34	0.4099	1.67	0.4525	2.00	0.4772	2.66	0.4961
1.35	0.4115	1.68	0.4535	2.02	0.4783	2.68	0.4963
1.36	0.4131	1.69	0.4545	2.04	0.4793	2.70	0.4965
1.37	0.4147	1.70	0.4554	2.06	0.4803	2.72	0.4967
1.38	0.4162	1.71	0.4564	2.08	0.4812	2.74	0.4969
1.39	0.4177	1.72	0.4573	2.10	0.4821	2.76	0.4971
1.40	0.4192	1.73	0.4582	2.12	0.4830	2.78	0.4973
1.41	0.4207	1.74	0.4591	2.14	0.4838	2.80	0.4974
1.43	0.4236	1.76	0.4608	2.18	0.4854	2.84	0.4977
1.44	0.4251	1.77	0.4616	2.20	0.4861	2.86	0.4979
1.45	0.4265	1.78	0.4625	2.22	0.4868	2.88	0.4980
1.46	0.4279	1.79	0.4633	2.24	0.4875	2.90	0.4981
1.47	0.4292	1.80	0.4641	2.26	0.4881	2.92	0.4982
1.48	0.4306	1.81	0.4649	2.28	0.4887	2.94	0.4984
1.49	0.4319	1.82	0.4656	2.30	0.4893	2.96	0.4985
1.50	0.4332	1.83	0.4664	2.32	0.4898	2.98	0.4986
1.51	0.4345	1.84	0.4671	2.34	0.4904	3.00	0.49865
1.52	0.4357	1.85	0.4678	2.36	0.4909	3.20	0.49931
1.53	0.4370	1.86	0.4686	2.38	0.4913	3.40	0.49966
1.54	0.4382	1.87	0.4693	2.40	0.4918	3.60	0.49984
1.55	0.4394	1.88	0.4699	2.42	0.4922	3.80	0.49992
1.56	0.4406	1.89	0.4706	2.44	0.4927	4.00	0.49996
1.57	0.4418	1.90	0.4713	2.46	0.4931	4.50	0.49999
1.58	0.4429	1.91	0.4719	2.48	0.4934	5.00	0.49999
1.59	0.4441	1.92	0.4726	2.50	0.4938		
1.60	0.4452	1.93	0.4732	2.52	0.4941		

Critical Values of the Student's t Distribution

Degrees of freedom k	Significance level p (**Two-sided** test)					
	0.1	0.05	0.02	0.01	0.002	0.001
1	6.31	12.7	31.82	63.7	318.3	637.0
2	2.92	4.30	6.97	9.92	22.33	31.6
3	2.35	3.18	4.54	5.84	10.22	12.9
4	2.13	2.78	3.75	4.60	7.17	8.61
5	2.01	2.57	3.37	4.03	5.89	6.86
6	1.94	2.45	3.14	3.71	5.21	5.96
7	1.89	2.36	3.00	3.50	4.79	5.40
8	1.86	2.31	2.90	3.36	4.50	5.04
9	1.83	2.26	2.82	3.25	4.30	4.78
10	1.81	2.23	2.76	3.17	4.14	4.59
11	1.80	2.20	2.72	3.11	4.03	4.44
12	1.78	2.18	2.68	3.05	3.93	4.32
13	1.77	2.16	2.65	3.01	3.85	4.22
14	1.76	2.14	2.62	2.98	3.79	4.14
15	1.75	2.13	2.60	2.95	3.73	4.07
16	1.75	2.12	2.58	2.92	3.69	4.01
17	1.74	2.11	2.57	2.90	3.65	3.96
18	1.73	2.10	2.55	2.88	3.61	3.92
19	1.73	2.09	2.54	2.86	3.58	3.88
20	1.73	2.09	2.53	2.85	3.55	3.85
21	1.72	2.08	2.52	2.83	3.53	3.82
22	1.72	2.07	2.51	2.82	3.51	3.79
23	1.71	2.07	2.50	2.81	3.49	3.77
24	1.71	2.06	2.49	2.80	3.47	3.74
25	1.71	2.06	2.49	2.79	3.45	3.72
26	1.71	2.06	2.48	2.78	3.44	3.71
27	1.71	2.05	2.47	2.77	3.42	3.69
28	1.70	2.05	2.46	2.76	3.40	3.66
29	1.70	2.05	2.46	2.76	3.40	3.66
30	1.70	2.04	2.46	2.75	3.39	3.65
40	1.68	2.02	2.42	2.70	3.31	3.55
60	1.67	2.00	2.39	2.66	3.23	3.46
120	1.66	1.98	2.36	2.62	3.17	3.37
∞	1.64	1.96	2.33	2.58	3.09	3.37
Degrees of freedom k	0.05	0.025	0.01	0.005	0.001	0.0005
	Significance level p (**one-sided** test)					

Table of Values χ^2. Pearson Distribution

Degrees of freedom k	Significance level p					
	0.2	0.1	0.05	0.02	0.01	0.001
1	1.642	2.706	3.841	5.412	6.635	10.827
2	3.219	4.605	5.991	7.824	9.210	13.815
3	4.642	6.251	7.815	9.837	11.345	16.266
4	5.989	7.779	9.488	11.668	13.277	18.467
5	7.289	9.236	11.070	13.388	15.086	20.515
6	8.558	10.645	12.592	15.033	16.812	22.457
7	9.803	12.017	14.067	16.622	18.475	24.322
8	11.030	13.362	15.507	18.168	20.090	26.125
9	12.242	14.684	16.919	19.679	21.666	27.877
10	13.442	15.987	18.307	21.161	23.209	29.588
11	14.631	17.275	19.675	22.618	24.725	31.264
12	15.812	18.549	21.026	24.054	26.217	32.909
13	16.985	19.812	22.362	25.472	27.688	34.528
14	18.151	21.064	23.685	26.783	29.141	36.123
15	19.311	22.307	24.996	28.259	30.578	37.697
16	20.465	23.542	26.296	29.633	32.000	39.252
17	21.615	24.769	27.587	30.995	33.409	40.790
18	22.760	25.989	28.869	32.346	34.805	42.312
19	23.900	27.204	30.144	33.687	36.191	43.820
20	25.038	28.412	31.410	35.020	37.566	45.315
21	26.171	29.615	32.671	36.343	38.932	46.797
22	27.301	30.813	33.924	37.659	40.289	48.268
23	28.429	32.007	35.172	38.968	41.638	49.728
24	29.553	33.196	36.415	40.270	42.980	51.179
25	30.675	34.382	37.652	41.566	44.314	52.620
26	31.795	35.563	38.885	42.856	45.642	54.052
27	32.912	36.741	40.113	44.140	46.963	55.476
28	34.027	37.916	41.337	45.419	48.278	56.893
29	35.139	39.087	42.557	46.693	49.588	58.302
30	36.250	40.256	43.773	47.962	50.892	59.703

Critical Values F For The Fisher Distribution
(k_{in}- number of degrees of freedom of within-group variance, k_b – number of degrees of freedom of between-group variable), level of significance p=0.05

k_{in} / k_b	1	2	3	4	5	6	7	8	12	24	∞
1	161.4	199.5	215.7	224.6	230.2	234.0	237.0	238.9	243.9	249.0	254.3
2	18.51	19.00	19.16	19.25	19.30	19.33	19.36	19.37	19.41	19.45	19.50
3	10.13	9.55	9.28	9.12	9.01	8.94	8.88	8.84	8.74	8.64	8.53
4	7.71	6.94	6.59	6.39	6.26	6.16	6.09	6.04	5.91	5.77	5.63
5	6.61	5.79	5.41	5.19	5.05	4.95	4.88	4.82	4.68	4.53	4.36
6	5.99	5.14	4.76	4.53	4.39	4.28	4.21	4.15	4.00	3.84	3.67
7	5.59	4.74	4.35	4.12	3.97	3.87	3.79	3.73	3.57	3.41	3.23
8	5.32	4.46	4.07	3.84	3.69	3.58	3.50	3.44	3.28	3.12	2.93
9	5.12	4.26	3.86	3.63	3.48	3.37	3.29	3.23	3.07	2.90	2.71
10	4.96	4.10	3.71	3.48	3.33	3.22	3.14	3.07	2.91	2.74	2.54
11	4.84	3.98	3.59	3.36	3.20	3.09	3.01	2.95	2.79	2.61	2.40
12	4.75	3.88	3.49	3.26	3.11	3.00	2.92	2.85	2.69	2.50	2.30
13	4.67	3.80	3.41	3.18	3.02	2.92	2.84	2.77	2.60	2.42	2.21
14	4.60	3.74	3.34	3.11	2.96	2.85	2.77	2.70	2.53	2.35	2.13
15	4.54	3.68	3.29	3.06	2.90	2.79	2.70	2.64	2.48	2.29	2.07
16	4.49	3.63	3.24	3.01	2.85	2.74	2.66	2.59	2.42	2.24	2.01
17	4.45	3.59	3.20	2.96	2.81	2.70	2.62	2.55	2.38	2.19	1.96
18	4.41	3.55	3.16	2.93	2.77	2.66	2.58	2.51	2.34	2.15	1.92
19	4.38	3.52	3.13	2.90	2.74	2.63	2.55	2.48	2.31	2.11	1.88
20	4.35	3.49	3.10	2.87	2.71	2.60	2.52	2.45	2.28	2.08	1.84
22	4.30	3.44	3.05	2.82	2.66	2.55	2.47	2.40	2.23	2.03	1.78
24	4.26	3.40	3.01	2.78	2.62	2.51	2.43	2.36	2.18	1.98	1.73
26	4.22	3.37	2.98	2.74	2.59	2.47	2.39	2.32	2.15	1.90	1.69
28	4.20	3.34	2.95	2.71	2.56	2.44	2.36	2.29	2.12	1.91	1.65
32	4.15	3.30	2.90	2.67	2.51	2.40	2.32	2.25	2.07	1.86	1.59
36	4.11	3.20	2.86	2.63	2.48	2.36	2.28	2.21	2.03	1.82	1.55
40	4.08	3.23	2.84	2.61	2.45	2.34	2.25	2.18	2.00	1.79	1.51
60	4.00	3.15	2.76	2.52	2.37	2.25	2.17	2.10	1.92	1.70	1.39
∞	3.84	2.99	2.60	2.37	2.21	2.09	2.01	1.94	1.75	1.52	1.00

Limits Of The Confidence Interval For The Median

The values in the table represent the ranks in the ascending ordered list of observations, which accounts for about 90.95%, or the 99% confidence interval for the median of the population based on one sample.

Example: the 99% confidence interval for the population median calculated on the sample of 56 observations is determined by observations with ranks 18 and 39.

Sample size	Confidence probability		
	90%	95%	99%
6	1;6	1;6	-
7	1;7	1;7	-
8	2; 7	1;8	1;8
9	2; 8	2; 8	1;9
10	2; 9	2; 9	1; 10
11	3;9	2; 10	1; 11
12	3; 10	3; 10	2; 11
13	4; 10	3; 11	2; 12
14	4; 11	3; 12	2; 13
15	4; 12	4; 12	3; 13
16	5; 12	4; 13	3; 14
17	5; 13	5; 13	3; 15
18	6; 13	5; 14	4; 15
19	6; 14	5; 15	4; 16
20	6; 15	6; 15	4; 17
21	7; 15	6; 16	5; 17
22	7; 16	6; 17	5; 18
23	8; 16	7; 17	5; 19
24	8; 17	7; 18	6; 19
25	8; 18	8; 18	6; 20
26	9; 18	8; 19	7; 20
27	9; 19	8; 20	7; 21
28	10; 19	9; 20	7; 22
29	10; 20	9; 21	8; 22
30	11;20	10; 21	8; 23
31	11;21	10; 22	8; 24
32	11; 22	10; 23	9; 24
33	12; 22	11;23	9; 25
34	12; 23	11;24	10; 25
35	13; 23	12; 24	10; 26
36	13; 24	12; 25	10; 27
37	14; 24	13; 25	11;27
38	14; 25	13; 26	11; 28
39	14; 26	13; 27	12; 28

Sample size	Confidence probability		
	90%	95%	99%
40	15; 26	14; 27	12; 29
41	15; 27	14; 28	12; 30
42	16; 27	15; 28	13; 30
43	16; 28	15; 29	13;31
44	17; 28	16; 29	14; 31
45	17; 29	16; 30	14; 32
46	17; 30	16; 31	14; 33
47	18; 30	17; 31	15; 33
48	18; 31	17; 32	15; 34
49	19;31	18; 32	16; 34
50	19; 32	18; 33	16; 35
51	20; 32	19; 33	16; 36
52	20; 33	19; 34	17; 36
53	21;33	19; 35	17; 37
54	21; 34	20; 35	18; 37
55	21; 35	20; 36	18; 38
56	22; 35	21;36	18; 39
57	22; 36	21;37	19; 39
58	23; 36	22; 37	19; 40
59	23; 37	22; 38	20; 40
60	24; 37	22; 39	20; 41
61	24; 38	23; 39	21;41
62	25; 38	23; 40	21;42
63	25; 39	24; 40	21;43
64	25; 40	24; 41	22; 43
65	26; 40	25; 41	22; 44
66	26; 41	25; 42	23; 44
67	27; 41	26; 42	23; 45
68	27; 42	26; 43	23; 46
69	28; 42	26; 44	24; 46
70	28; 43	27; 44	24; 47
71	29; 43	27; 45	25; 47
72	29; 44	28; 45	25; 48
73	29; 45	28; 46	26; 48
84	34; 51	33; 52	30; 55
85	35; 51	33; 53	31;55
86	35; 52	34; 53	31; 56
87	36; 52	34; 54	32; 56
88	36; 53	35; 54	32; 57
89	37; 53	35; 55	32; 58
90	37; 54	36; 55	33; 58

Sample size	Confidence probability		
	90%	95%	99%
91	38; 54	36; 56	33; 59
92	38; 55	37; 56	34; 59
93	39; 55	37; 57	34; 60
94	39; 56	38; 57	35; 60
95	39; 57	38; 58	35; 61
96	40; 57	38; 59	35; 62
97	40; 58	39; 59	36; 62
98	41; 58	39; 60	36; 63
99	41; 59	40; 60	37; 63
100	42; 59	40; 61	37; 64

The Limits Of Confidence Intervals For Relative Frequencies

In the column headings - numerators;
in the line headings - denominators.
Example: If 5 patients out of 30 have the complication, the relative frequency is 0.167, and the 95% confidence interval is [0.056 0.347].

Denominator	Numerator						
	0	1	2	3	4	5	6
1	.000 .975	.025 1.00					
2	.000 .842	.013 .987	.158 1.00				
3	.000 .708	.008 .906	.094 .992	.292 1.00			
4	.000 .602	.006 .806	.068 .932	.194 .994	.398 1.00		
5	.000 .522	.005 .716	.053 .853	.147 .947	.284 .995	.478 1.00	
6	.000 .459	.004 .641	.043 .777	.118 .882	.223 .957	.359 .996	.541 1.00
7	.000 .410	.004 .579	.037 .710	.099 .816	.184 .901	.290 .963	.421 .996
8	.000 .369	.003 .527	.032 .651	.085 .755	.157 .843	.245 .915	.349 .968
9	.000 .336	.003 .482	.028 .600	.075 .701	.137 .788	.212 .863	.299 .925
10	.000 .308	.003 .445	.025 .556	.067 .652	.122 .738	.187 .813	.262 .878
11	.000 .285	.002 .413	.023 .518	.060 .610	.109 .692	.167 .766	.234 .833
12	.000 .265	.002 .385	.021 .484	.055 .572	.099 .651	.152 .723	.211 .789
13	.000 .247	.002 .360	.019 .454	.050 .538	.091 .614	.139 .684	.192 .749
14	.000 .232	.002 .339	.018 .428	.047 .508	.084 .581	.128 .649	.177 .711
15	.000 .218	.002 .319	.017 .405	.043 .481	.078 .551	.118 .616	.163 .677
16	.000 .206	.002 .302	.016 .383	.040 .456	.073 .524	.110 .587	.152 .646
17	.000 .195	.001 .287	.015 .364	.038 .434	.068 .499	.103 .560	.142 .617
18	.000 .185	.001 .273	.014 .347	.036 .414	.064 .476	.097 .535	.133 .590
19	.000 .176	.001 .260	.013 .331	.034 .396	.061 .456	.091 .512	.126 .566
20	.000 .168	.001 .249	.012 .317	.032 .379	.057 .437	.087 .491	.119 .543
21	.000 .161	.001 .238	.012 .304	.030 .363	.054 .419	.082 .472	.113 .522
22	.000 .154	.001 .228	.011 .292	.029 .349	.052 .403	.078 .454	.107 .502
23	.000 .148	.001 .219	.011 .280	.028 .336	.050 .388	.075 .437	.102 .484
24	.000 .142	.001 .211	.010 .270	.027 .324	.047 .374	.071 .422	.098 .467
25	.000 .137	.001 .204	.010 .260	.025 .312	.045 .361	.068 .407	.094 .451
26	.000 .132	.001 .196	.009 .251	.024 .302	.044 .349	.066 .394	.090 .436
27	.000 .128	.001 .190	.009 .243	.024 .292	.042 .337	.063 .381	.086 .423
28	.000 .123	.001 .183	.009 .235	.023 .282	.040 .327	.061 .369	.083 .410
29	.000 .119	.001 .178	.008 .228	.022 .274	.039 .317	.058 .358	.080 .397
30	.000 .116	.001 .172	.008 .221	.021 .265	.038 .307	.056 .347	.077 .386

Denominator	Numerator						
	7	8	9	10	11	12	13
1							
2							
3							
4							
5							
6							
7	.590 1.00						
8	.473 .997	.631 1.00					
9	.400 .972	.518 .997	.664 1.00				
10	.348 .933	.444 .975	.555 .997	.692 1.00			
11	.308 .891	.390 .940	.482 .977	.587 .998	.715 1.00		
12	.277 .848	.349 .901	.428 .945	.516 .979	.615 .998	.735 1.00	
13	.251 .808	.316 .861	.386 .909	.462 .950	.546 .981	.640 .998	.753 1.00
14	.230 .770	.289 .823	.351 .872	.419 .916	.492 .953	.572 .982	.661 .998
15	.213 .734	.266 .787	.323 .837	.384 .882	.449 .922	.519 .957	.595 .983
16	.198 .701	.247 .753	.299 .802	.354 .848	.413 .890	.476 .927	.544 .960
17	.184 .671	.230 .722	.278 .770	.329 .816	.383 .858	.440 .897	.501 .932
18	.173 .643	.215 .692	.260 .740	.308 .785	.357 .827	.410 .867	.465 .903
19	.163 .616	.203 .665	.244 .711	.289 .756	.335 .797	.384 .837	.434 .874
20	.154 .592	.191 .639	.231 .685	.272 .728	.315 .769	.361 .809	.408 .846
21	.146 .570	.181 .616	.218 .660	.257 .702	.298 .743	.340 .782	.384 .819
22	.139 .549	.172 .593	.207 .636	.244 .678	.282 .718	.322 .756	.364 .793
23	.132 .529	.164 .573	.197 .615	.232 .655	.268 .694	.306 .732	.345 .768
24	.126 .511	.156 .553	.188 .594	.221 .634	.256 .672	.291 .709	.328 .744
25	.121 .494	.149 .535	.180 .575	.211 .613	.244 .651	.278 .687	.313 .722
26	.116 .478	.143 .518	.172 .557	.202 .594	.234 .631	.266 .666	.299 .701
27	.111 .463	.138 .502	.165 .540	.194 .576	.224 .612	.255 .647	.287 .681
28	.107 .449	.132 .487	.159 .524	.186 .559	.215 .594	.245 .628	.275 .661
29	.103 .435	.127 .472	.153 .508	.179 .543	.207 .577	.235 .611	.264 .643
30	.099 .423	.123 .459	.147 .494	.173 .528	.199 .561	.227 .594	.255 .626

Denominator	Numerator					
	14	15	16	17	18	19
1						
2						
3						
4						
5						
6						
7						
8						
9						
10						
11						
12						
13						
14	.768 1.00					
15	.681 .998	.782 1.00				
16	.617 .984	.698 .998	.794 1.00			
17	.566 .962	.636 .985	.713 .999	.805 1.00		
18	.524 .936	.586 .964	.653 .986	.727 .999	.815 1.00	
19	.488 .909	.544 .939	.604 .966	.669 .987	.740 .999	.824. 1.00
20	.457 .881	.509 .913	.563 .943	.621 .968	.683 .988	.751 .999
21	.430 .854	.478 .887	.528 .918	.581 .946	.637 .970	.696 .988
22	.407 .828	.451 .861	.498 .893	.546 .922	.597 .948	.651 .971
23	.385 .803	.427 .836	.471 .868	.516 .898	.563 .925	.612 .950
24	.366 .779	.406 .812	.447 .844	.489 .874	.533 .902	.578 .929
25	.349 .756	.387 .789	.425 .820	.465 .851	.506 .879	.549 .906
26	.334 .734	.369 .766	.406 .798	.443 .828	.482 .857	.522 .884
27	.319 .713	.353 .745	.388 .776	.424 .806	.460 .835	.498 .862
28	.306 .694	.339 .725	.372 .755	.406 .785	.441 .814	.476 .841
29	.294 .675	.325 .706	.357 .736	.389 .765	.423 .793	.457 .821
30	.283 .657	.313 .687	.343 .717	.374 .745	.406 .773	.439 .801

203

Altman's nomogram

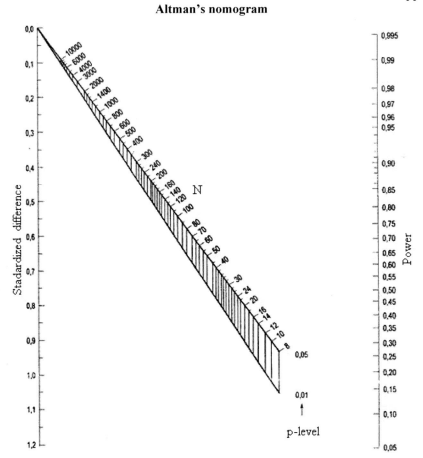

CONTENT